THE THINDERELLA
SYNDROME

THE THINDERELLA SYNDROME

A PRACTICAL GUIDE TO INDIVIDUALIZED PERMANENT WEIGHT LOSS

Dennis Gage, M.D., F.A.C.P.

With a Foreword by Dr. Richard Janof

PUBLISHING DIVISION OF PERMANENS LLC

The opinions expressed herein are solely those of the author. Readers should seek the advice of their personal physicians before starting any new diet or medical program.

Author photo by
Selwyn Fund Prestige Photography, Inc.
Cover Design by www.innervisiondesign.net

Contents

"Dr. Gage has written a pithy and insightful text on weight loss, easy to read with meaningful observations and readily implemental measures to counteract the results of our sedentary lifestyles."

—Marina Kurian, M.D.

"Dr. Gage avoids the fad diet mentality and espouses a sensible scientific approach to achieving and maintaining weight loss. He provides numerous imaginative techniques, based on his own successful weight loss and that of many of his patients, to promote healthy eating and exercise habits."

—Allan Geliebter, Ph.D.

"Losing weight is like having sex. Once you've reached your goal, it's orgasm all the way."

—Susan Faye Meltzer

"I am a private trainer at the Sports Club L.A. in New York. Through Dr. Gage and Dr. Janof, I have dropped almost 30 pounds in a healthy and safe way. Just by manipulating my diet and consistent weight training and cardio, my goals have been accomplished."

—Andrew Bogate

"Read this book and find out how Dennis Gage and his staff saved my life."

—William Scott

"When I first met Dr. Gage, I was overweight, lethargic, and had blood sugar and adrenal problems that adversely affected my quality of life. Only through very hard work, getting my body balanced using supplements and thyroid medication, and cleaning up my diet was I able, at age thirty-eight, to finally feel and look the way I've always wanted. You can't just sort of do this; you must make a *lifestyle* commitment and change everything as you know it. If you are sick enough and want your life back, you'll do it and see how great it feels to be happy with the body you have. This year I competed for the first time and won the title 'Ms. Figure Empire State' and came in second place at the national championships. It took me thirty-eight years to get it together. Now that I have, I'll never go back. I could never have imagined this level of health ten years ago."

—Tara Marie Segundo

"At last I have found a realistic way to lose weight and keep it off. The ability to change my lifestyle habits has truly permitted me to change my life permanently."

—Katiana Harrison

"After a long struggle I have lost 115 pounds in one year. I look forward to more loss. I started at 435 pounds and will continue to 204 pounds, my goal. Dr. Gage and Dr. Janof are my support system for a lighter life."

—David Atkins

"Dr. Gage has shown me how to 'Live' a diet. After doing fad diet after fad diet after fad diet, I have finally been able to lose weight and keep it off permanently, by using Dr. Gage's phenomenal techniques."

—Daisy Negron

"Dear Dr. Gage:

"I feel so very fortunate to have you as my specialist physician. Your expertise, knowledge, and dedication have positively impacted my life. Losing over 160 pounds is as unbelievable to me as was surviving at 450 pounds. In acknowledging this accomplishment, I share with you my success and look forward to a continued gainful year under your guidance and supervision.

"Thank you so very much."

—Sincerely,

Marcella

FOREWORD

BY DR. RICHARD JANOF

HAVING treated many obese patients in my nutritional practice, I have come to realize how important an inherent behavioral change in lifestyle is necessary to combat the continual bombardment of Western civilized foods upon the body. Daily I see the ravages of obesity—perhaps it's the poorly controlled diabetic or the arthritic patient who no longer is able to walk at age forty—but in all cases we see multiple examples of obesity-related diseases.

Dr. Gage demonstrates how everyday lifestyle is the crux to whether an individual is successful at weight maintenance or whether that person will fall into the "Thinderella Syndrome" and regain weight back and then some.

Does anyone actually think Cinderella would have fit into that glass slipper if she were forty pounds overweight? Forget about it. The royal beau might have been looking more favorably upon those two ugly stepsisters who were at least thin!

But then again, that is a fairy tale and so is expecting a handsome prince or anyone else to save you from your dilemma. If being overweight is your problem, there are no magic solutions, no princes, and no Fairy Godmothers. But there is a way out and it can be fun. Everyone has a natural balance to their body, a native weight, and when that balance is overturned the body reacts by overeating, with the attendant lifestyle changes, less activity, less interaction with people, emotional reactions of anger, shame—the list grows and grows.

Dieting and failing bring on added problems and a subsequent loss of faith. These problems escalate and soon you find yourself looking for that prince or a magic bullet in diet scams, programs, shakes, gum, pills, anything to stop the mounting pounds. When none of these work, you really do feel like that poor little scullery maid.

Dr. Gage in his no-gimmick way explains in a stepwise fashion what really must be done to lose weight and maintain a healthy weight throughout life. He simplifies the process of behavior modification by breaking down lifestyle changes into small, easy-to-do pattern changes. Patients are then encouraged because they see they can change without the stress and pressure induced by traditional "crash diets."

However, Dr. Gage goes further and explains why patients "yo-yo" and how they can prevent this cycle from occurring. His defensive-eating-style patterns ensure the patient of a permanent, individualized, long-lasting weight loss and maintenance success.

In my twelve years of teaching Dr. Gage's behavioral techniques, I have seen firsthand the ability of a patient to permanently change his or her eating style and then be successful in long-term weight control. I have also seen the fruitless weight loss that occurs on traditional fad diets. I see clearly that when I am able to convince obese patients to follow the road map of the "Three R's" (Realization, Regimentation, and Reorientation), they are able to transform their lifestyles, their weights, and their lives with permanent success. I am convinced there is no alternate way to succeed. There is no magic pill. Thinderella is really only a figment of the imagination. The real you is defined by the lifestyle you practice. So go ahead and live your diet and be you for a lifetime, instead of Thinderella for a day.

—Dr. Richard Janof, D.C., C.D.N., C.D.E.
Chiropractic Medicine
Clinical Nutrition
Certified Diabetic Educator

PREFACE

AT last—here is a book on dieting that takes a sane, realistic approach to the methodology of weight loss. Dr. Dennis Gage is an expert in obesity and has treated literally hundreds of patients successfully over a twenty-two-year period using his "behavior-modification-defensive-eating-style approach."

Dr. Gage claims that there is not really one kind of obesity, but rather, multiple types. Every patient has a group of individually different eating patterns that in the end cause a gain in weight beyond the norm. Therefore, Dr. Gage customizes his approach to weight loss for each reader.

Unlike other books that describe single methodologies as a mode of weight loss, such as: "carbohydrate loading," "starvation," and "formula dieting," Dr. Gage offers a custom-made group of behavioral interventions that, when applied, will work for each individual. Through his theory of the three R's of behavior modification: Realization, Regimentation, and Reorientation, he describes what is involved in taking back control of one's eating lifestyle.

But Dr. Gage goes beyond a successful methodology for healthy weight loss. He puts forward a group of techniques for weight maintenance that he calls "defensive eating style." Through continued patterning and awareness, the patient is able to maintain a healthy goal weight indefinitely, and, if weight gain does occur, Dr. Gage describes his "red alert" warning system that restores control back to the patient. Never again should a patient "yo-yo." The message is clear: if you must diet at all, then do it the right way and keep it off permanently.

End the "Thinderella Syndrome" for good. Forget about magic potions and fairy tales. Greater than 97 percent of patients on other diets regain the weight they have lost. Recent scientific evidence has shown that "yo-yo" dieting is as unhealthy as never dieting to begin with. So look at a methodology that is realistic, healthy, permanent, and finally, successful:

Dr. Gage's Defensive-Eating Style

Before and After Photographs

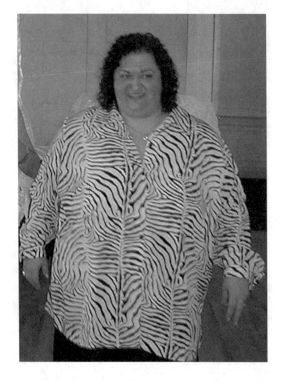

"I've lost 190 pounds in 18 months. Through Dr. Gage's guidance, I've been living each day with the diet; I'm not just on a diet. I'm proud of myself now and very grateful to Dr. Gage."

—Gloria Argueta

Turn the page to see the new me.

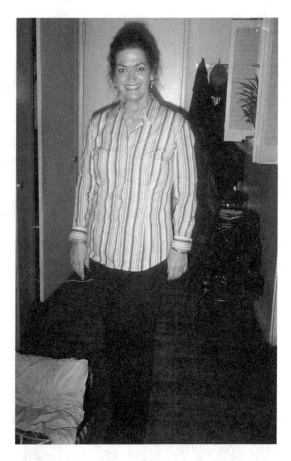

Gloria Argueta

Acknowledgments

I have many people to thank for making this book possible but especially so to my loving wife, Madeline, who put up with me throughout the eight years of writing and rewriting the book, a large part on vacation! She also typed the entire manuscript!

To my children, Jacob, Aaron, Rachelle, and Joshua, who spurred me on and said, "So where is the book already?"

To my patients who inspired me to complete the work for their sake.

I finally thank G-d for permitting me to finish the work. I hope it will help many individuals. Yes, a special note of thanks to Ms. Margaret McGovern for the much-needed editing and to my good friend and colleague, Dr. Richard Janof.

I

DR. GAGE'S STORY

I T was a warm summer day. I had been a resident for less than two months at Mount Sinai Hospital. I remember the time. We had recently had a hurricane that hit the New York area and I was busily learning my new rotation. I was driving a Mustang "fast back sedan." On the way back from working at Elmhurst Hospital, the car was going across town at Ninety-seventh Street when suddenly out of the blue, another car passed the light at Lexington and Ninety-seventh careening into the right passenger side of my car. It all happened so fast—but things appeared to be happening in slow motion in almost a surreal way. I saw shattered glass flying, the car being dragged down the street. I was stunned and thought it was all over!

My lip was bleeding profusely, and my glasses had vanished. With my foggy sight, it was apparent that the passenger side of the vehicle was gone, crumpled up metal was bundled up next to my right leg. The heap that was once my car stood motionless. I cried out for help, but it was as if the world had gone on vacation. The driver of the other vehicle had fled. I learned later that he did not have a license and had been arrested several times for DWI. I noticed then several neighborhood kids. I cried out for help, but they went running.

Finally there were police and ambulance sirens. The driver door of my vehicle was opened in a crunch. I kept crying out that I was bleeding, but then I spontaneously stood up out of the car. A police officer handed me my glasses, slightly battered but still functional. He said, "Don't worry, just a gash on your lip. I think you will be fine." These were the comforting words I heard. I gathered my composure. What next?

"Let the attendants take you to the emergency room." I arrived at the Mount Sinai Hospital Emergency Room. The nurse took my vital signs, weight—190 pounds, height—five foot ten, blood pressure slightly high 140/92. I was described as "mildly obese." My lip was cleaned up and I seemed otherwise okay but I was asked to stay several hours for observation. I thought to myself, *am I really obese? Is my blood pressure going up?* After all I was just twenty-seven years old. *How bad a shape can I be in?* I had no broken bones or internal injuries. At that point I did not realize it, but this incident was to be the major motivator in changing my behavior and patterns forever.

I left the Emergency Room in time for a late bite to eat. I met up with a close friend and told him the whole story. "Let's check out the car," he said. My friend thought I was really lucky. He said, "That seatbelt saved your life. Look at that wreck, you must have been hit at forty miles per hour plus." We surveyed the car. It was a goner. Even the insurance company agreed. But as for me I was about to embark on a new lifestyle. I asked my friend, "Do you think I am fat?" He answered, "Well, I wouldn't say fat, but maybe a bit overweight."

I retired for the night, thinking of the days' events. Serendipitously, I was about to start a rotation in Rheumatology (the specialty dealing with joint diseases). The professor was a relatively young attending physician, who was an excellent teacher. But it wasn't the teaching that got me all excited. It was his own enthusiasm and obsession with jogging. He was training for the New York Marathon, and he would tell me how he successfully completed a six-mile or twelve-mile run. "Why don't you just join New York Road Runner's Club?" he asked. "As a doctor you could volunteer at the New York Marathon finish line and help out."

It sounded exciting to me. The marathon was less than two months away, and my professor was hoping to just finish the race. I decided to try it out, that is, jogging. I bought a pair of Nike sneakers. All excited I headed out to Central Park. I was going to run around the bridle path, a distance of

1.55 miles. I stretched out a bit, and off I went. However, after running about a two-block distance or so, I was huffing and puffing, almost gasping for air. I pushed harder, but at about one-third the distance I needed to stop. I just walked the rest of the way, disgruntled and in disbelief that a twenty-seven-year-old person could be this out of shape! But I didn't give up. The very next day I returned to the same spot. I stretched and this time slowly jogged almost at a walking pace. With some difficulties I made it around the 1.55 mile track. I was now a bit more enthusiastic, so for the third day in a row, I went for it, completing the full track. Somewhat sore, I was feeling proud.

I awoke the next morning with excruciating pain in my knees. I could not bend them or go up and down stairs without pain. I managed to go down the subway stairs and get to my rheumatology rotation. My professor knew right away. "You have a bad case of chondromalacia patellae (irritation from the knee cap). Well, take these two Motrin and let me show you the exercise to do in order to stretch your quads. Don't run for a few days and you should then be fine." I took his advice, but ended up being out of commission for ten days. Over those ten days, I had read several manuals on running and foot care. I was committing myself to doing this thing right! I would stretch more often, go at a slower pace, and run every other day instead of daily. I also realized that some form of calorie restriction would help, so I decreased my bread and dessert intake.

Foolishly, I had increased my cheese intake, thinking this was healthy, but I learned at a later time how much fat was in cheese. By the time my professor ran the marathon, I was persistently running 1.5 miles three to four times per week. My professor finished the marathon in four and a half hours. He was exhausted and it took him one month to recuperate. I always thought he pushed too hard, so six months went by and I increased my mileage to three miles four times per week. I suffered through several more injuries (the diseases of excellence as runners know it), calcaneal bone bruise, plantar fascitis, and a knee strain, but my persistence and slow training methods were turning into a true lifestyle, and I proceeded cautiously with my exercise. Indeed at this point, I had lost twenty pounds, weighing in at 170 pounds and I felt so much better. People were noticing the weight loss, and I started socializing more with Latin dance class and calisthenics. Yes, still more exercise.

Over the next four months, I became a true exercise fanatic. I bought the runner's watch and timer, the best shoes, and logs for tracking my time. I was truly enjoying the run, listening to music, at this point, six miles was a breeze. I would get out from my residency, sign out patients, and immediately go for my jog around all of Central Park (about six miles). I found this very relaxing and invigorating, even after being on-call with sometimes less than three hours' sleep. I would look forward to the run.

I was taught by my early days of running that even if I am exhausted with little sleep, I get so much out of the run that it is very much a positive reinforcer. Unlike some of my friends who feel that they *must* exercise, I feel I want to exercise. Call it the "runner's high." I call it a positive motivator. Two months before marathon time, I was 142 pounds, able to run six miles in forty-five minutes, and I had run a half-marathon and several 10K races. I had my eye on the marathon and couldn't get in. One of my buddies who was accepted got injured, so I just took his place. I finished the 1979 Marathon in four hours and fifteen minutes and proceeded to run the 1980 New York Marathon in three hours and thirty-one minutes. My weight was stable at 140 pounds. I also remember biking to work for six months. This was probably set off by the New York subway strike at the time.

Interestingly, my calorie intake was at the highest level ever. I needed approximately four thousand calories a day to support my high activity level. In those days carbohydrate loading was in. I would put away boxes of pastas without putting on a pound. My waist size went from a 37 to a 32. I even went down one shoe size and ring size. It was truly a metamorphosis; but lifestyles do change. I never ran another marathon because of time restraints, but I continued to run five to six mile runs for years.

My next big lifestyle occurrence was marriage. Fortunately, my wife also liked to exercise, so little change in my patterns were necessary, but then along came our first child, Jacob. Wow! What a lifestyle change. For one, I ate with my wife's cravings through the pregnancy and at some point had regained six to seven pounds of the forty-five pounds lost.

Secondly, from the time my son was born, family patterns

changed dramatically. We were home most days, and dinner became the most important meal of the day. I immediately realized that I would have to reassess my lifestyle situation. I kept food records for approximately two to three weeks and realized what was going awry. I was now eating a large lunch at the office and a large dinner at home. Unlike before my wife's pregnancy when there was only one major meal, lunch. There were now two. I also realized that with being increasingly busy in the office, I had less and less time to eat. Indeed there was no longer a lunchtime, let alone a lunch hour, and I instead found myself wolfing down a pint of Chinese fried rice, here, a doughnut there, etc. The most reasonable answer to me was that if I can't enjoy the meal, why waste calories? I decided to initiate my first major behavioral defensive pattern since losing my original weight seven years earlier.

Little did I know that I was about to practice "strict avoidance technique" and "banking and preplanning." Well, I started out by eating three to four fruits per day. The technique appeared to be working. I lost two to three pounds, but would this pattern stay? Only time would tell. As it turned out, I did have a slight lapse after vacation that year. It took me six weeks to get back on a "fruit for lunch" pattern, but now at the time of writing this book, the technique is approaching its four-teenth year and still works like a charm.

Once again I must say, this technique has lasted not simply because of my forcing myself to eat fruit, but because of several positive reinforcers working simultaneously. These include the ability to eat fruit neatly and swiftly between patients, that is convenience, and its low calorie content, permitting me to bank some calories into the weekend. I also learned to spend on my high-calorie foods when I had more leisure time.

As the years have passed on, I realized I had several other challenging lifestyle changes; some with my family growing bigger, others with moving and commuting. At one point I needed to tune up my techniques and realized that my enjoyable run had been squeezed down to two and a half to three miles two to three times per week. I saw there were the usual time restraints, so I simply committed to increasing my run by ten minutes. This brought my calorie- burning capacity up to four and a half miles three times per week. I felt that extending the run as opposed to increasing frequency of run was more time efficient, and this worked. At another point I analyzed the salad dressing that I was using. It was a light diet dressing, but contained thirty calories per tablespoon. I found a substitute dressing at ten calories per tablespoon, using three to four tablespoons five times per week, I saved quite a number of hidden calories.

People to this day still ask me how I keep the weight off? And how I have done it for so many years? It has now been twenty years since I lost my original (pre-dieting) weight! My answer is, "You live a diet, you don't do a diet." My second answer is, "There is very little difference in dieting and maintaining a healthy weight." The patterns and styles required for one are generally still required for the other. You must remember the three R's of Behavior Modification which you will soon read about—this is "working" the third R, Reorientation.

II

Obesity—Man's Modern Way to Diseases— the Diseases of Opulence and Success

YEARS ago, obesity was a disease only of the wealthy and prosperous, the few. The common people, "peasants," ate what was available; grain, rice, beans—they worked long hours and burned calories readily. Their diets were low in fat and high in fiber. Some people like the Pema Indians and some nomad tribes lived a semi-starvation existence, living off the land. Despite this, these people were relatively healthy. They were lean and fit. Infections, such as pneumonia, measles, and small pox, were the cause of their demise.

On the other hand, we had wealthy people: bankers, land-owners, and aristocrats who had the ability to afford the "good life." They ate beef, cheeses, wine, rich baked goods, and more. They were sedentary, sitting at their desks, having everything brought to them on a "silver platter." They gained weight easily and in general developed obesity-related diseases, such as heart attack, gout, gallstones, and Pickwickian's Disease (Sleep Apnea Syndrome).

Now there are a lot of examples in history of the above stark contrast of societies' groups. The Russian Revolution's soldiers at the front ate common food: grain, fiber, fruit, whatever was available. They were lean, mobile, and relatively healthy. Their major risk was getting shot or getting an infection. The generals and officers, the backfront, on the other hand, had lots of beef, milk, cheese, etc. They were safe behind the front, but their myocardial infarction rate was high. They were in poor physical shape. This was the way it was even at the end of the nineteenth century.

But something happened—with the mechanization and modernization of agricultural techniques and the ability to preserve and store foods and produce foods at cheaper prices, things went "topsy turvy." Food became plentiful and was readily available. This occurred first in the United States and Western Europe, but food abundance by the 70s, 80s, and 90s spread into Third World Nations.

Fast foods were in—eating a hot dog or burger became the mainstay. Grabbing your Coke and a hot dog was easier than getting a prepared salad. People left the farm environment and came to industry and service jobs. They sat at desks at the same time when modern mechanization came into being. We had the elevator, automobile, and escalator. This first mechanical revolution affected adults by decreasing their energy output and "saving them time" at the cost of increasing obesity and weight gain.

The second mechanical revolution was just as bad, if not worse. It was the insidious growth and popularity of the television, the computer, video games, and wireless technology.

People no longer needed to walk or move. Everything became automatic, and unfortunately, even our children stopped playing ball and outdoor activities. They became "couch potatoes" and "computer addicts." They sit now in front of TV, videos, and computers, using the remote control to change the channel. They are more sedentary than ever!

Thus came the deadly epidemic of obesity. I say deadly, for as I will tell you later, obesity causes a whole host of diseases. At this point obesity is only second to cigarette smoking as a leading cause of death, and in fact it could seriously challenge the number one position as the obesity epidemic worsens and spreads throughout the world. Hints of the epidemic were apparent a decade ago. Generally lean, healthy people, such as the Polynesian Islanders and the U.S. Pema Indians began dramatically increasing weight.

Why? Because food from fast-food chains and processed foods reached these people. These were people used to eating off the land. Suddenly, processed foods, cakes, candy, burgers, fries, were all introduced at once. Genetically these Third World nation groups were well equipped to eat natural foods from the ground: fruits, berries, fish, etc. Now the environment produced a sabotaging fat, high sugar, high salt diet. The result was devastating— the Pema Indians have one of the highest diabetes rates in the world. Fifty to sixty percent of them have diabetes and high cholesterol. Gallstones have increased dramatically in this population. A natural health disaster all created by the refined products of modern man. The same thing was happening to Polynesian people in whom obesity used to be considered a good thing for the rulers: kings and queens. It has now devastated the health of the rest of the people. Similar stories have occurred in almost all areas of the world. Perhaps they have suddenly become "Westernized."

Here in the United States, the government has declared a diabetic emergency. The epidemic in the U.S. is quite severe. Startling statistics now indicate an obesity rate of approximately forty percent, with an overweight rate pushing beyond sixty percent of the general population. Diabetes- Type 2, almost unheard of until adulthood, is now breaking loose in our obese teens and youngsters. These young patients are requiring medication to control the diabetes. The rate of diabetes is directly related to one's weight, even a ten percent increase in weight nearly triples the risk of Type 2 Diabetes. Patients with severe obesity increase their risk by fifty to sixty times the norm.

Presently there are estimated to be eighteen million diabetics in the U.S., about seven million going undiagnosed. The rate of dysglycemia (prediabetes) has not even been considered. This involves the abnormal blood sugar that occurs three to seven years before diabetes develops. Perhaps another thirty to fifty million people are affected.

It was 1992 when Kaplan, et al. wrote his clinical paper called "The Deadly Quartet." This paper helped us understand how obesity was directly related to several disease states and death. As you will see in my chapter on nutrition (chapter VII), I describe a continuum of foods with unhealthy diet being the most insulin stimulating. Kaplan described scientifically a cascade of events that occurs when someone gains weight and becomes obese. The metabolically active fat is deposited in the gut, both inside and outside the body " the proverbial apple shape."

Now these fat cells become resistant to the effect of your body's own insulin. This is called Insulin Resistance and is thought to be the central "theme" that causes all the problems. Insulin Resistance causes your body to put out even more insulin to overcome the problem, and this stimulates several things. For one, you increase the amount of triglycerides or fat in the blood: "This is how excess carbohydrates are stored." The increase in triglycerides is accompanied by an increase in cholesterol. Both these substances accelerate the atherosclerotic process, which causes plaques to develop in the arteries of vital organs, such as your heart and brain. Eventually, this leads to blockage. Clinically, you have a heart attack or a stroke. The above can be illustrated as follows:

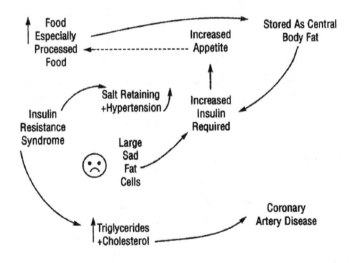

Don't worry too much about the details of this diagram, just understand the far-reaching effect that obesity has on your health. There is a tremendous cascade effect so that obesity is related to a whole host of diseases. Note that the high insulin levels will cause your body to retain salt and thus increase the risk of hypertension. The above ingredients are thus appropriately named the "Deadly Quartet," for they are the recipe that induces fatal heart attack and stroke. If things are not bad enough, there are still a whole host of diseases associated with obesity. Several female cancers appear more likely in the obese: uterine and breast cancer may occur more frequently because the age at which a woman starts to menstruate is earlier the heavier they are. Obese girls are starting to menstruate at age nine to ten and therefore have a longer time exposed to estrogen cycle.

Colon and gallbladder cancers appear to be more common in the obese. Prostate cancer in men appears to be more common in the obese. Other diseases seen in the obese include sleep apnea. This disease occurs frequently in the obese and causes the individual to momentarily stop breathing while he or she sleeps. This occurs numerous times during the night. The individual develops sleep deprivation at night and never gets quality-time sleep. The long-term result is increased blood pressure in the lungs with subsequent thickening of the heart. These individuals are predisposed to "sudden death syndrome." These individuals are also involved in five percent of fatal auto accidents, for they frequently fall asleep at the wheel since they are so sleep deprived at night.

Gallstones are more apt to occur in the obese. All med students know of the four Fs of gallstone disease that predispose patients to gallstone disease: Female, Fat, Forty, and Fertile. However, gallstone risk is also increased in the obese male. Osteoarthritis is still another obesity-related illness. Osteoarthritis—most of us think of an elderly male or female, cane in hand, hobbling down the street when we think of osteoarthritis. So when my thirty-six-year-old obese female patient was brought in by wheelchair, it seemed odd to the other patients in the waiting room. She weighed 275 pounds and had been obese since her teens. She weighed perhaps 175 pounds by age fifteen. In her twenties, she developed increased pain and decreased mobility, but everybody blamed her "slowing down" on her weight. She weighed about 250 pounds by age thirty, and at this point was seen by a specialist who told her to "lose weight." She never did because unbeknownst to the doctor, she already had significant degeneration of both of her knee joints. At age thirty-six, when she could barely walk, her parents insisted that she go to an orthopedic specialist who, with x-rays, diagnosed end-stage osteoarthritis of both knees.

She came to my office because the orthopedic surgeon wanted to replace both knees surgically and he required that she get her weight down below 200 pounds. Stories like this one are unfortunately not uncommon in my obese patients. Many of them develop premature osteoarthritis in the knees and hips at an early age. Sadly, these patients lose the ability to get around, and further they lose the all-important ability to burn calories by walking.

Many a patient has come into my office complaining of increased weight over one or two years. They say, "But, Doc, I am actually eating less." I answer, "But, patient, you are also walking less." The patient's comment: "Well, yes, my knees ache and I can't go more than one to two blocks a day." Well, yes, ten years ago, I successfully dieted and exercised by walking two to three miles per day. It is at this point when I review with these patients the all-important calorie-burning capacity of walking. "Well," I say, "two miles a day equals 240 calories burned a day, is equal to 15.8 pounds per year. Not walking equals fifteen pounds gained per year. But since you ate a bit less, you only gained ten pounds per year." Thus, osteoarthritis is one of those double whammy diseases that create not only the painful disease but also the vicious cycle of decreased activity yielding more sedentary lifestyle, yielding continued eating, yielding increased weight with further degeneration of joints and further decrease in activity and so on. This downward spiral is one of the most difficult to break since it requires increased caloric restriction, as exercise is obviously limited to swimming and upper body activity. Finally, obese individuals are more accident prone due to their weight and are poor surgical risks.

So we look at the obese world today. The poor and middle class are the obese and sick; they suffer a malnutrition "overabundance and overindulgence." They are not physically fit, for they watch TV forty hours a week and work desk jobs in front of computers. They are more stressed, eat quicker, and eat more. Their children watch TV, eat, and play video games. They also suffer this malnutrition and lack of physical fitness. Ironically it is the middle upper class and wealthy who have become more health conscious. They spend more money to get fresh vegetables, fruit, and fresh foods. They join health clubs and hire trainers to force themselves to exercise. They are weight conscious.

Unfortunately, they also indulge in the good life. Many think leanness, health, and beauty can be simply bought, but most have been proven wrong. It takes lifestyle change and permanent commitment to maintain a healthy weight and body. Hopefully, by utilizing the techniques in this book, this will be an obtainable goal.

III

MEDICAL CURES OR JUST PATCHWORK

MANY patients in my practice have recently become more complacent regarding healthy weight. Because of the numerous cures and treatments that are now out there for diabetes, high cholesterol, and lipid abnormalities, they believe they just need to "take a pill for this and a pill for that." The end result has been less emphasis on prevention and healthy weight loss and more emphasis on medical "patchwork" treatment.

I call it "patchwork" because most of the modern medicines don't get to the root of the problem. Instead, medicines treat an end result = disease. If a patient becomes diabetic, he or she is more apt to ask for a pill that will treat the sugar than ask for a healthy preventative treatment, which would include diet and exercise. The end result is a biochemical mixture of medications that are trying to stimulate normal physiologic function to the extreme. These medications are man-made and all have potential side effects, both short and long term.

Let's look at an example of one of my patients who is more interested in medication treatment of diabetes. The patient—a 215-pound, five-foot-nine-inch male—came into the office

with high blood sugars. Though diet was initially spoken of
and instruction given, the patient deemphasized the diet and
emphasized the wonderful new armada of medicines available
to treat diabetes. He started initially on one pill that stimulated his body to produce more insulin. This brought the sugar
down, but he proceeded to gain fifteen pounds of weight and
came in one year later with a normal blood sugar and a weight
of 230 pounds. He remained inactive and not interested in diet.

He eventually needed two more medications, one for
cholesterol elevation and another medication to get his blood
sugar down, as it had crept up over the preceding years. At
this point he weighed 242 pounds, had two medications for
diabetes, and one medication for cholesterol. He complained
of fatigue and increased water in the legs. He was placed on a
"water pill" and a potassium supplement pill. He then developed leg cramps and some increased shortness of breath. He
came into the office one spring morning and though his blood
sugar and cholesterol were well controlled, his weight was up to
256 pounds and he was tired. Blood tests also revealed elevated
liver tests. He asked for my advice, and I told him, "Let's stop
all these patchwork cures and get back to basics. If you buy a
car, you don't want one with souped-up parts that have been
added on to keep it running. You want a well-tuned-up engine
with original parts."

He finally saw the light, and we started him on a motivator-
type diet with formula, fruits and vegetables at 1,400 calories,
and a multivitamin. We immediately stopped three medications,
and he lost twelve pounds in two weeks. Blood tests revealed
improvement in liver function and not only that, the cholesterol
and sugar were in excellent control.

After two months on a motivator-type diet, the patient

went through behavioral patterning and training. He had lost forty pounds of weight and was down to 216 pounds, just about the weight at which he needed medication #1 to begin with. But amazingly, he was now exercising three to four times per week, eating rather healthy, and doing daily food records. He felt much less tired and was invigorated. He eventually brought his weight down to 195 pounds and was able to get off all the medication. His body was healthier and ran like a smoothly tuned engine.

So much for medication. It should be common sense that if one can treat and prevent illness through natural means, then this is the obvious choice. The problem is everybody wants the "magic pill." Again the "Thinderella Syndrome" strikes. Patients say, "Give me a pill to make me thin." Now people say, "Well, if I can't be thin, just give me a pill to keep me healthy." As one can see, this kind of magical thinking is self-defeating. It puts all hope in medicines and the doctor but takes away participation of the all-important patient. Patients want to be taken care of, but they don't want to take care of themselves. This leads to patients being treated solely for the goal of correcting a medical condition as we illustrated above. This seldom works.

Instead the patient must take an active role in obtaining health and preventing disease. When this occurs all modalities to wellness are used and medications take a secondary but still important role in treatment. Whenever a patient arrives at my office with an obesity induced illness, I tell him or her there are two pathways that one can follow. The first pathway, the more difficult, will involve lifestyle change, calorie restrictions, some exercise but probably less medicine. You, the patient, will be thinner, feel better, and look better. You will be prone to less obesity-induced diseases. You, the patient, will have more control and say as to what happens to your body and life.

The second choice involves medication treatment, adding medicines as needed to the regimen. This is the easier path. You just need to take your medicines. Your weight may go up. You will still be prone to other obesity-related conditions, especially if you are gaining weight. You may need more medications over time. You, the patient, will give up your control and depend on medication monitoring and doctor-prescribed treatments. Almost always when patients are told upfront of the long-term consequence of a treatment, they will go with the first choice.

IV

THE ROAD TO
BEHAVIORAL CHANGE

INTRODUCTION

AFTER twenty-two years of treating patients with obesity, I have developed a group of parameters that I believe help define the disease, its treatment and, finally, the all-important methodology of keeping the disease in remission. Simply put, the ability to lose weight and keep it off depends on lifestyle change via behavior modification techniques. I say "simply" because "it is easier said than done."

Most diets concentrate on only one pattern or technique. Patients enforce or regiment themselves to a specific pattern, for example, "eat only vegetables." The patient is enthusiastic initially because he gets control over his eating style. He loses weight and is happy. He pays attention and adheres to the diet. However, over time, boredom sets in, weight loss slows, or perhaps the patient is sabotaged, goes off the diet, gains back the weight and "yo-yo's," only to try the next fad diet and repeat the same activity.

What is involved in the process called behavior mod are three very basic patterns that must be traversed and accepted.

These are the three R's of behavior mod, namely, Realization, Regimentation, and Reorientation.

Realization involves the ability to accept and not run away from the basic facts. The food record for the most part will measure this parameter. A patient who runs away from the record is generally considered resistant. He may be denying that there is a problem with food to begin with or his priorities may be skewed with the desire to lose weight really lower down on the "totem pole" of desires than he initially expected. Alternately, many patients associate anxiety, depression, and loss of control with food intake. They may have been conditioned to fear food, for they associated it with weight gain, loss of self-esteem, loss of control, etc.

This being the case, it is much easier to understand why they hide from looking at the food record as it is a confession in detail of the so-called "crime." A bank robber would never think of filming his heist. He is usually secretive and wants to appear incognito. Some patients are perfectionists. If the job can't be done right, they won't do it at all! This type of patient will write records out if they represent the correct intake of food and if all is in order. The minute the patient feels the record is not up to par, i.e., transgression has occurred— the food record ceases to exist. These patients see things in black and white or "all or none."

Thus, realization involves acceptance of the eating behavior. The patient must feel comfortable recording all ingesting data. To do this, he must first be "de-sensitized" from the high anxiety of the act of eating itself. Patients in our office are encouraged to write all ingestions down. They are praised and rewarded for reporting everything. This, despite the quality and quantity of the food.

Food is not considered good or bad. No ethical correlation is given. The process of de-sensitization is a difficult one. Dr. Claire Weeks in her book, *Hope and Help for Your Nerves,* describes several components to de-sensitization that are involved in any action. First, there is facing and not running away from the fact itself. Second, accepting the ingestion as an occurrence and not emotionally fighting over the worthlessness or worthiness of it. Third, is to float or not create waves. This involves not building up undue or unnecessary emotions about the particular ingestion. Fourth, is repeating the process with practice over time. When successful, the patient will feel comfortable describing all ingestions to the therapist and the first phase—Realization—will be well on the way to being conquered.

Regimentation is defined in the dictionary as "to organize rigidly especially for the sake of regulation or control." Control over food intake is obviously of prime concern. Ultimately it is the acceptance of ways to control food intake in some manner that will yield a permanent weight loss.

Regimentation of eating habits encompasses the basic tangible eating techniques, whether it be nutritional regimentation, like eating a specific food, such as vegetables, or a technique, like sitting down while one is eating. There is still initiation of a habit that will control the ultimate intake of food. Regimented physical activity looks at the other end of the spectrum. Control of burning calories guarantees weight loss to the exact extent of the particular activity.

Most food fad diets out there use a specific single regimentation technique. Usually, it is the eating of one food type or the pattern of eating that is changed. A patient will adhere to the regimentation and do well; however, the underlying habit is not ultimately accepted as a lifestyle change. The habit will be extinguished. Old habits will ensue, and the patient will "fall off the wagon" and regain the weight.

Because most fad diets ask for such extreme change, they are, from the onset, doomed to failure. For example, though most of us can eat grapefruit for one or two or maybe three months, it would be the rare patient who continues to eat grapefruit as the mainstay of his or her diet for life. On the other hand, many of us can accept the concept of eating grapefruit for breakfast as a permanent pattern change knowing that there is still some variety for lunch and dinner. Thus, the greater the change, the less likely it is to be successful in the long run. This is why behavior mod works best by making small-step pattern changes that can be practiced, managed, and accepted without overwhelming the patient.

Manageability is a cognitively defined term. Some patients can take bigger steps than others. I usually advise my patients to set very small goals or steps at first so that they can be successful managing them. Once there is confidence in these tasks, patients are encouraged to try more complex ones.

You can see now that the Realization and Regimentation phases of behavior mod are well-traveled courses. Almost all dieting patients have gone through an awareness of maladaptive eating and have then initiated a regimented pattern diet. So why then are there such dismal results with less than three percent of dieters permanently keeping weight off while most of us just yo-yo up and down the scale? The answer to this question lies in the third and most important phase of behavior mod. It is the "R" of Reorientation. This word spells out the cognitive acceptance or rejection of the diet or diet technique. And 97 percent of dieters fail to "reorient."

Most individuals are successful in Realization and

Regimentation and lose varying amounts of weight, but then something happens. There is a slowing down in weight loss. There is fatigue and boredom in one's pattern of dieting. But most important, the changes made to initiate the diet are either too drastic, too punishing, too unrealistic, and suddenly negative thinking appears.

Why does this happen? There are several reasons: First, people tend to pick unrealistic, drastic techniques because these generally yield the most significant and dramatic weight loss rates. These techniques are supported by the "all-powerful scale," which at the beginning of the diet gratifies the patient with the pounds going down. The positive support there becomes the scale and as long as the scale shows weight going down at the right rate, the patient remains highly motivated. Because the scale is the only supporter to motivate these patients, it also may become the biggest form of sabotage.

We all know patients who have lost 50, 60, even 100 pounds only to falter down the road! Suddenly the scale says "Sorry, no weight loss this week;" or worse yet "one to two pounds gained!" Patients now feel defeated, frustrated, disillusioned, and abandoned. They develop that dreaded condition, "Scalitis," in which the only thing that counts is the almighty scale.

They try more drastic techniques, hoping to see just one more pound down. Ultimately, these patients fail, for they have had only one goal, and that is to see the number on the scale go down. They have unfortunately lost the initial concept of why they were dieting. They have become slaves to the scale whereby pounds down equals success and pounds up or unmoving equals failure. They cease dieting. Angry, frustrated, defeated, and depressed, they try to put blame on their slow metabolism, the rotten diet that was "no good to begin with," or worse, on themselves, saying "I am just no good or not worthy to lose this weight."

This negative condition not only destroys the diet but sets the patient up for further failure spirals. We all know those patients who have yo-yo'ed up and down several times, only to try another diet next year. Ultimately they come to expect failure because, after all, "that's what happens whenever I diet."

They remain slaves to the scale, never learning what true reorientation is all about. Remember, to diet is to "change lifestyle" and not just to lose weight. Weight loss per se is only a by-product of lifestyle change. Lifestyle changes must occur piecemeal and slowly via behavioral changes that are positively supported by new activities. The succeeding chapters will describe many regimentation techniques, but none of them will work if they are not positively supported as permanent long-term goals. The ability to accept a pattern and positively support it for a lifetime is what reorientation is all about.

Another factor that comes into play to make reorientation difficult is the sheer force of nature. As one loses weight, several things happen to the metabolism. Nature perceives weight loss as a threat to the organism, and when weight loss is significant, metabolic rates decrease. Nature tries to protect the organism, and one of the ways to do this is to preserve calories.

Thus, when metabolic rate goes down, fewer calories are burned and it is harder to continue losing weight. When one compares the metabolic rate of two people—one who has always weighed 190 pounds to a person who was initially 250 pounds and has lost 60 pounds, now weighing 190 pounds—the latter person will have a metabolic rate that is perhaps 20 to 30 percent less than the former. Call this unfair but from nature's standpoint, it is a survival mechanism.

Our survival over millions of years (if you believe Darwinian theory) is based on the ability to utilize fuel most efficiently. Those cave people who could not slow their metabolic rates down and had no food available, perished. The cave folk who could slow down their metabolic rate were more likely to survive until there was food available. So blame this situation on your ancestors, but realize they didn't have huge grocery stores and fancy restaurants until recently.

To reorient one's behavior is to truly accept a habit as permanent. This requires us to positively support the habit. We notice what happens when a habit is enforced by a sheer number on the scale. Inevitably, weight loss plateaus and the positive reinforcement is extinguished or, in the worse case scenario, replaced by negativism. When one chooses a habit, it must fit one's lifestyle and receive support for other reasons.

When I practice my pre-planning technique in the office, I take into consideration my lifestyle (non-stop busy), my orientation toward healthy eating, and my desire to eat out on the weekends. So when I eat four to five pieces of fruit during the day, it presents to me, convenience. I can eat between seeing patients without wasting time. It is healthy, I get in my fruit groups, and it is relatively low in calories so that I can bank and save calories for the weekend. It also presents to me a method of defending my healthy weight—something that is really crucial for long-lasting weight control to occur.

Reorienting one's behavior is thus an acceptance of new habits, but not for the sole cause of seeing the scale go down. By taking the pressure off one's ability to lose weight on the scale, patients are able to concentrate on the true task at hand: changing eating style. When one develops confidence in these techniques, they will know that the weight loss follows.

When my patients practice behavior mod for the first time, I challenge them with an interesting task. I ask them to trust those food records and not look at the scale number at all. Since the scale is completely eliminated, they must put all their faith in the food records, which now become the major prognosticator of what will happen to their weight. In other words, I am giving the patient realistic tasks that can be practiced at different paces and degrees.

The result is that the patient has the ability to see change occur in a spectrum of stages or "gray zones." He or she realizes that weight loss is not just "all or none." The scale is black and white. I either lose the pounds successfully or gain the pounds and am defeated. But behavioral techniques have gray shades. You can have varying degrees of success measured on a food record and never be a failure. There are only varying shades of success. When more changes are permanently made, the more intense the shade of gray, but notice when one accepts the "gray zone scale" and falters with one technique, one merely falls back to a slightly lighter shade of gray compared to the "all or none" weight loss ideal. When one falters, one goes from white to black or vice versa. I will devote an entire chapter to the "gray zone" because within its many shades lie the answers to defensive eating and permanent weight loss.

V

WHY A FOOD RECORD?

THE Food Record is a blueprint of one's eating behavior, but it measures far more than this. Food records test one's willingness to diet. In a sense, it is a test of priorities. Patients who are willing to do them are generally more motivated and willing to make changes. Patient's food records, like a builder's blueprint, give a clear, precise picture of how a patient's eating habits interact with his or her environment in everyday lifestyle.

Certainly, you would never think of building or remodeling a home without a blueprint. Just picture the builder saying, "Don't worry. I have a clear picture in my mind exactly where the kitchen should be!" Because one's eating habits may be in disarray, many patients try to avoid being aware of them. They would rather eat and "hide the evidence."

This very important theme will come up time and time again. Since overeating and maladaptive eating are considered by both patients and society to be "bad," keeping records is like "confessing one's sins to the priest or doctor." In other words, the patient looks at overeating and food records as a negative bad deed. They run away from the evidence instead of facing the facts. Patients must understand that behavior mod will only work if it is positively supported by them. Therefore, the record must be looked at as a map, with the road to success going through rough territory. The record can be looked on positively if the patient sees it as a means of *controlling* intake. Control is a potent weapon, a positive force that can put things in order.

The record outline is of great importance. Though all records are of help, the more defined the eating behavior is, and the more the parameters and interactions that are considered, the easier it becomes to shape a particular behavior. Consider at this time several record formats.

Our first format will be writing out records longhand in a notebook. Here, a certain amount of information is recorded very much the way one books an appointment with a colleague. The description is put down in a log form, and the patient is able to refer to this book and see past ingestions.

The second format takes on a more shaped behavior pattern. Here the food is described in detail, a calorie assignment is now given to this particular food, and the patient notes that a particular goal is being practiced.

The third type of food record, which is a very interactive one, will best shape healthy eating behaviors. Here, a number of parameters are described, the time it takes the patient to eat the food, the place at which the patient eats the food, the activity that the patient is involved in at the time, the mood, degree of hunger, etc. Notice that although the complexity of the record increases, so does the shaping and descriptiveness of how one interacts with the environment. Thus, the more information we know about the ingestion, the more we can learn on how to change it and restructure it. Thus, the shaping of the behavior is the key to why behavior mod will work on one's diet as compared to other fad diets.

Most fad diets have you practice an enforced lifestyle. The weight loss may occur, but there is no structure supporting this weight loss. Think of being on top of a building with a shaky infrastructure. The slightest wind or temperature change may collapse the entire building. Now, with behavior mod, picture securing and intensely fortifying this building floor by floor. Though the process may be slower, the building is far more secure and you can safely sit on the top floors without worrying. Thus, a food record that breaks down each pound of eating behaviors step by step will permit one to build a much sturdier building than one that does not.

Unfortunately, it is this very strength of behavior mod that causes the most problems. Patients are looking for that "quick fix." Patients truly believe that the faster the pounds roll off, the better the diet. Patients just don't have patience! They want their diet to miraculously occur. It is this very type of thinking that will never permit the true shaping of behaviors to occur.

A REAL CASE STUDY

Patient R.J. came to my office weighing 240 pounds. She had lost weight many times over the years, only to yo-yo back up again. We discussed the importance of re- cord-keeping, and she initially kept some records. But with time, she stopped doing them. Despite this, she came for her weekly visits and was actually doing well with weight loss of approximately three pounds a week. She was enthusiastic and nearly euphoric. She related to me weekly in a verbal way how she could eat vegetables and grains without problems and how easy it was to keep to this kind of a diet.

Despite continued discussions on how she had not yet attempted to change her lifestyle habits, or address long-term change, she resisted talking about it or taking action on it. About five months into the diet, with nearly a forty-pound weight loss, she began missing appointments and was lost to follow-up. About one year later, she came to the office and, somewhat embarrassingly, admitted that she never really did attempt to make the changes that we discussed a year ago.

Don't expect sturdy skyscrapers to pop out of the ground like magic. It takes guided work, using a clearly defined blueprint. In our next section, we will define the actual blueprint so that we can begin to redesign a new lifestyle.

BLUEPRINT FOR A NEW LIFESTYLE

In this section, I will guide you through the various parameters we can measure. I will use the most detailed blueprint. Those patients who desire to can limit themselves to the more simple formats; however, remember the more one records, the more things that can be shaped and changed in one's behavior.

1. Speed of eating. How fast does one eat in a particular ingestion? Here, one must record the time at the start and at the completion of the ingestion. Consider a cessation of eating for fifteen minutes or greater to signify the end of eating. For example, if you have dessert one hour after your meal, consider it another ingestion.

2. Place of eating. For example, don't just say "at home"; describe the room, kitchen, bedroom, etc. At work, describe the exact place of eating; at the desk, in the work cafeteria, or at a conference table.

3. Describe the position. Are you sitting, standing or lying down?

4. Associated activity. What are you doing at the time that you are ingesting the food? Are you working, reading, talking, listening to music, watching TV, etc.?

5. Alone or with whom. Be as specific as you can.

6. Mood. Try to describe your feelings at the time you are about to eat. Are you rushed, depressed, are you happy? Do you feel tense and anxious, or do you feel relaxed?

7. Amount of food. Be very critical here. Either measure with a cup or a scale. You may also read off amounts from packaged goods. If in doubt, try to estimate. Practice your visual acumen on the size of foods by first estimating the size and then officially weighing the food. Most patients grossly underestimate their portion sizes.

8. Describe the food in detail. Don't just say one doughnut, say one medium-sized glazed doughnut. Don't just say a bagel, say a large-sized raisin bagel with butter.

9. Estimate calories. Don't let calories intimidate you. Don't try to memorize the calorie content of each food. Think of foods as fitting into basic food groups. The American Diabetes Association has a booklet that describes this in detail. This book is based on calorie food groups and not on individual foods. Once you understand a particular group, you may extrapolate calories to all the member foods in a group. Even if you are not in the mood to look up calories, place down your estimates. When you respond in a group or in a one-on-one session, you

can review these estimates and see how reasonable you were.

10. Cognitive consequences of the ingestion. Describe your feelings after eating—was it considered a "cheating eat" and did you feel guilty? Was food "not deserved?" Was the food well planned out, etc.?

11. Weight graph. Graph out your week-by-week weight. This is a great motivator and will help you follow your progress. Don't look at a particular week, but rather, as your stockbroker looks at the trends, you are to look at the overall trends in your weight loss. Though many of the dots on the graph may go up a pound or two here and there, if the overall trend on the graph is on a downward slope, you are making progress. This type of methodology will help you focus away from the week-to-week weight loss changes that one often gets hung up on.

12. Measurements. You may wish to follow the waist and hip measurements graph. These tend to change less with water weight change and therefore tend to be more representative of what is really happening to your body.

13. Monitor your physical activity. Many patients keep great food records, but tend to ignore or grossly simplify physical activity records. One should break down physical activity into daily routines or physical activity in everyday lifestyle and into another category called leisure activity. Thus, you can monitor daily lifestyle changes by monitoring the miles you walk around during your typical day. This is best done by wearing a pedometer. Most are reasonably priced

between $15 and $20 and will add a tangible dimension to your daily activity. The pedometer is also a great motivator.

14. <u>Leisure activity.</u> This activity should be monitored by type of activity, intensity, and duration. For example, if you are jogging, describe it as jogging moderately (10 mph) times thirty minutes. By breaking down the activity in this fashion, one has at least several parameters that can be worked on.

VI

TANGIBLE BEHAVIORAL TECHNIQUES

SLOWING DOWN

HAVING grown up in New York City, I have frequently encountered some of the "most rushed people" in the world. New York City's pace is lightning fast. Unfortunately, food intake can also latch onto a hectic lifestyle, and we therefore have some of the speediest eaters right here in New York. What is wrong with rapid eating? Why should we slow down the pace of eating?

Well, for one thing, most people believe that the act of eating should be an enjoyable process. Eating slowly permits one to taste the food more distinctively. After all, gulping a hot dog down on the street corner while rushing to a business meeting may be filling, but did that person really taste and enjoy the ingestion, or was it just an "ingestion of habit." Like, "Oh, it is 1:30 P.M., if I don't grab this now, I won't get a chance to eat again till dinnertime." This patient barely tasted the food. Indeed, outside of the habit of eating "lunch," there was no other pleasure attached to this ingestion. In fact, the patient, by eating too fast, probably got indigestion!

Now, compare this to going to the best French restaurant in town (an often-debated issue in itself). You sit down at a beautifully set table, candles, flowers and silverware, the music sounds in the background. The meal is served slowly and eaten slowly. The fireplace burns a red glow, with the sound of an occasional crackle. The food is beautifully presented. You savor every bit, eating slowly while talking to your closest friend. Your overall experience is very enjoyable.

Another reason to eat slowly is the obvious fact that given certain time limits, only a specific amount of food can be eaten. The quicker one eats, the more calories consumed within this time frame. If one is able to slow down the speed of eating, there are simply fewer calories consumed. As an example, let's assume you get a half-hour off at lunchtime. You decide to have a frankfurter. Depending on how fast you are, you can eat anywhere from one hot dog up to fifty (a record held by Nathan's 2001 Fifth of July contest). Any technique that slows you down will therefore cause fewer calories to be ingested.

A third and very important reason for slowing down your eating is to permit your own body's physiological functions to take hold. We know from experiments that it takes approximately twenty minutes or so for the human stomach to tell the brain "it is full." This is done by intricate mechanisms that involve both hormonal and neuronal transmitters. The message is not completed until the twenty minutes pass.

I can vividly remember a case scenario when I was a medical intern at Mount Sinai Hospital in New York City. It was 11:30 P.M. and a bunch of us were sitting in the Klingenstein cafeteria having a midnight snack that consisted of leftover rice and beans and a few overdone hamburgers. Having not eaten since about 6:00 P.M. and having run around the hospital several times, we were all very hungry. As we signed out patients, we ate swiftly and persistently. About fifteen minutes into this giant snack, our beepers went off, a code 777 was on the way to the E.R. and was to arrive immediately.

We were all hungry, but we knew we would have to leave the meal to attend to the patient. We all reluctantly jumped up and took off for the Emergency Room. After waiting there about ten minutes, we found out the patient had ultimately been taken to nearby Metropolitan Hospital. We all went back to the cafeteria where about half our meal sat, but since it had been interrupted, we all felt stuffed and could not take another morsel. We blamed the loss of our appetite on the interruption. Indeed, the fifteen-minute gap in time permitted us to truly feel full. Our stomachs told our brains that it had enough to eat, and we were thus spared the excess calories. This scenario is common.

Most of us can remember times when our meals were interrupted for one reason or another. We think we are ravished, but we return to the meal only to realize that our appetites are now gone! The food suddenly does not look as appetizing. Indeed, we feel a bit cheated. Our hunger has been "robbed," and it is no longer pleasurable to eat, but it is this very mechanism designed by our own bodies that protects us from overeating. The key is to just give it time to "take hold."

Finally, there is another reason to slow down. It represents the ability to replace one habit with another more adaptive habit. Consider that all of us eat out of a feeling called "hunger." Hunger may be defined in many ways. Some people eat swiftly until they eat enough to become uncomfortably full. Others eat quickly to fill a void in the pit of their stomach or to ease a gastric discomfort, a feeling of acidity. Some people eat swiftly because they are rushed and feel they may not get another chance to eat later.

What is important is that all the above feelings may represent hunger, but the mode of squelching it tends to be maladaptive. Thus, we want to slow down the speed of eating to change over to a healthy and more adaptive habit, one that will satisfy our hunger and not overfeed us at the same time.

There are many methods that are around to slow down one's speed of eating. I would like to run through some of the classic ones and also mention a few "offbeat" methods. Putting utensils down is a well-accepted method of slowing down. If you watch people eat, you will see a certain style associated with different eating patterns. Many people, while eating, will prepare the next biteful of food while still chewing the previous mouthful. They are very efficient and have patterned their ingestion to go perfectly smooth; almost unconsciously, these people will begin cutting the next piece of food with the knife so that the fork or spoon arriving at their mouth is perfectly orchestrated.

What happens here is that the mechanism of eating has become perfectly efficient in speed of intake. Now when one puts down the utensils after an ingestion, there is a small delay in the speed of eating between each bite. The methodology used here involves putting all utensils or foods down until one swallows what is already in their mouth. The act of swallowing now signals one to pick up utensils or food for the next piece. In this technique, if you swallow food and you are still holding anything in your hand, you have goofed.

Of course, in the beginning of any new habit, you are bound to catch yourself going back to old habits and making mistakes, but with practice, the old habit will be extinguished.

This will occur only if you positively support the new behavior. Beware of compensating for a new habit.

One Patient's Way

Ms. R.H., a patient of mine, was at first having lots of success slowing down her eating style with the putting down of the utensil technique. But about three months into behavior mod, there seemed to be a loss of the importance in the slowing-down technique. R.H. was definitely still putting down utensils after each bite but was not sensing a slower style.

On further analysis, we found the culprit. She was compensating for the new technique by introducing another (negative) technique. She was taking "megabites" of food per mouthful, thus still eating as fast as she did before. It is not unusual to see sabotage techniques invade one's new eating style. Later on in the book, we will spend a great deal of time uncovering and dealing with sabotage events.

Smaller Pieces

The answer to R.H.'s problem was simple. We introduced another modification: cutting the food into smaller pieces in a purposeful fashion. This technique is relatively straightforward. The smaller pieces of food require an increased frequency of going to one's plate. Simply put, you can wolf down a hot dog in two to three bites (perhaps even slinging it down in one gulp!) or you can use a knife and fork and cut the hot dog into eight, ten, or even twelve morsels, savoring each biteful.

Chewing

Another slowing-down technique involves the actual

amount of counting of the number of chews per biteful of food taken. This technique brings to mind the fact that choking accidents in the U.S. kill 2,800 people per year. Though the technique of counting four, five, or six chews may turn some of us off to food, it has been useful to a number of my patients.

Sip of Fluids

Small sips of non-caloric beverage are another all-time favorite. This technique involves having a glass of water or non-caloric beverage beside your dish at the table. The patient takes one to two sips between every couple of bites of food. Clearly this habit has several advantages: for one, you get the benefit of filling up somewhat with fluid. This decreases hunger and satisfies you. We have all had the experience of drinking a carbonated beverage on a hot summer day, feeling totally "bloated," and losing at least in part, our appetite for solid food.

Secondly, sipping the fluid will automatically force one to put down utensils or food and thus increase the duration of the total ingestion. Finally, sipping fluids helps wash down the food, making the next bite more enjoyable (if you don't believe me, try eating a hard-boiled egg without any fluid).

Getting Up

Getting up from the table as a technique is not for everyone, but for the compulsive eater, it can be life-saving. The technique involves getting up from the table during mealtime, and it is helpful if you have a simple, positive task to carry out. That's why I usually combine this habit with "sips of fluid" technique.

Here is how it works: I tell the patient to take a small

juice-glass size of their favorite non-caloric beverage. No pitchers are allowed on the table. When the glass empties, the patient is forced to get up and pour more water or non-caloric beverage. This technique works well because the patient is clearly prepared and anticipates the need to get up during the meal. The patient, therefore, positively reinforces the habit.

In clear contradiction to this is getting up for nuisance reasons. Patient L.R., for instance, was practicing her slowing-down techniques. She related to me that she was always jumping up from the table to chase after her three-year-old who was constantly creating havoc during dinnertime. She would find this particularly irksome and would respond by forcefully eating even faster whenever she got a chance.

Therefore, this "getting up" technique was a negative one for her and was associated with rushed, unplanned bouts of having to leave an enjoyable meal. You can see that the above technique would lack the positive reinforcement necessary. Never practice a technique that ends up negatively impacting your behavior. If you catch yourself responding to a new habit by worsening your eating skills, you must extinguish the new habit. Make sure you are not simply resisting a new habit. That is, you may be angry with a new technique and respond negatively by rebelling, by acting out, and eating more. This falls into another form of sabotage.

To finish up the "slowing down" technique, I will mention a few other techniques that patients in my practice have used with success. Eating with chopsticks or with a small shrimp cocktail fork will slow you down in a mechanical sense. See how much longer it takes to eat a baked potato with a tiny shrimp fork. The trouble with this technique is that most of us gain technical expertise with these and therefore learn to eat quicker and more efficiently with them.

Finally, certain foods make us eat slowly. For example, hot soup cannot be gulped down without burning our mouths. We must blow on the soup to cool it down, and this takes time. Eating non-caloric foods, such as lettuce, salads, celery, etc., will slow us down because it takes more mechanical energy and more chomping to get these foods pre-digested and swallowed. Though our speed of eating doesn't change, our ability to get to the next caloric dish is actually slowed down.

PLACE OF EATING TECHNIQUE: EVERYTHING HAS ITS OWN PLACE

The goal here is to define very decisively the exact place for eating all your meals. Generally, one should be sitting down in a comfortable chair at a table that is set for the sole purpose of eating. The place should be very specific and kept the same. Many of you have several tables in your home, but only one should be defined as the place for eating. The ambiance of the environment is important, too.

We all know the enjoyment of eating in an expensive restaurant, the beautiful table setting, the atmosphere, the good service, and of course, the good food. The main event there is obviously to eat and the setting is appropriate. So make your table setting at home special so that it stands out. Get flowers for the table or a new place mat or tablecloth. This tends to emphasize the importance of place of eating. We want to highlight the enjoyment of eating your meal.

At work, things may be more difficult, but, again, a specific area should be defined. One should be comfortable, un-interrupted, and peaceful. If possible, a table and chair would be best, but at the desk, things are a bit more difficult. Try to clear a space at your desk so that you are not bothered with papers and work. Keep the phone off the hook so that your meal will be uninterrupted. It is obvious that emphasizing the place of eating makes one much more aware of the act of eating, but more than this, it is an attempt to break behavioral linkage that tends to cloud the eating ingestion.

We all know the problem that children have doing home-work and watching TV at the same time. The homework tends to be done slowly and in an inferior fashion. This is because the place for doing homework is not very conducive to study. TV steals the emphasis away from homework; thus in the end, the student has not fully paid attention to either work or, for that matter, to the TV program! Placing the student at a quiet, comfortable desk is obviously the appropriate place for homework. Things get done much more efficiently without interruption and usually in a much more concise manner.

This carries over to the eating arena also. There are numerous examples, but let us look at a case scenario first: Joe is the typical hard-working commuter. He gets up early, dressing hurriedly to make the 6:45 A.M. train. He rushes out of the house but quickly gulps down one vitamin pill and one glass of orange juice. At the train station, he grabs a newspaper, a bagel, and a cup of coffee. If he is lucky, he gets a seat on the train and reads his paper.

Many times the train runs off schedule, and he arrives at the office late. At work, he rushes in and out of meetings. He will grab a cinnamon Danish or two while at a conference. He may be pressured by the boss to produce quickly and on time. This rushing around gets him upset, and he frequently misses lunch. Instead, he grabs a doughnut off the secretary's desk with another cup of coffee. At 3:00 P.M., while passing a candy machine on the ground floor of his building, he picks up a Snickers bar. He tends to stay late at the office and falls asleep on the 6:35 P.M. train home.

When Joe arrives home, dinner is being prepared. To relax, he sits in the lazy chair watching TV and grabs a cluster of grapes. He finally eats dinner, commenting to his wife, "Gee, I'm starved. I had nothing all day and missed lunch!" After dinner, he plays with the kids a bit and grabs one or perhaps two of their Twinkies.

Joe came to my office one day wondering why he had put on forty pounds during the last two years. He told me he only ate sporadically and thought there must be something wrong with his metabolism. Joe's food records rapidly uncovered the culprits. There were: the 120-calorie juice, the 450-calorie bagel with 50-calorie cream and coffee, two Danishes of 350 calories each, one Snickers bar of 300 calories and finally, two Twinkies of 600 calories. And this was-n't even counting his one healthy meal at dinner.

Joe's problem was the diffuse spread of his eating technique. He ate at times and places not appropriate or conducive to good eating behavior. Most of his ingestions were overshadowed by work, a rushed atmosphere, tension, and a milieu that was certainly mundane. Indeed, the choice of food was very poor, and when I questioned Joe, he certainly did not enjoy most of these rushed meals.

Joe was a victim of eating out of place. Like the student with the homework, he never really paid great attention to the ingestion. Indeed, much of what was done was out of sheer maladaptive habit and not true hunger at all. Thus, we can appreciate that "place of eating" technique makes us much more aware of an ingestion. It underscores the fact that eating food in an appropriate setting should be the center of attraction. We can then enjoy the food for the pleasure of eating itself. And we can break the Pavlovian linkage of food to such typical scenarios as pretzels munched while watching TV in bed, grabbing a candy bar at the newsstand while waiting for a cab, or wolfing down a hot dog while cheering at a ballgame.

Yet there are some other behavioral attributes to the place of eating technique that warrant discussion—namely the decreased risk of ingesting ectopic foods. Clearly the fewer, more defined places we have to eat, the less food that is going to be ingested and the fewer calories consumed.

A Typical Scenario

Picture yourself in the family room watching an exciting television program. You may have ordinarily brought in some snack, like fruit or whatever, to eat during the program. Now if you practice a strict place of eating technique, you would need to leave the TV room, sit down at the designated table, and enjoy your snack there, missing some of the program. Most patients realize very shortly that they would rather continue watching the program and perhaps have the snack later. What usually occurs is that a certain percentage of snacking does not occur anymore at all. The reason behind this is that much of out-of-place eating occurs from sheer habit and not from true hunger.

When the behavior linkage between TV and food is broken, the food becomes less appetizing since true hunger never really existed. To further understand this, think of the popcorn scenario in the movies. What makes it enjoyable is the movie scene and atmosphere. Many times after dinner, people go to the movies and immediately get in line for popcorn, candy, or other snacks. Again, the linkage of movies and popcorn is so strong that I have had many patients tell me that without it they just cannot enjoy a movie. These people equate going to a movie as going to a movie and eating popcorn. Two separate habits are practiced so symbiotically that they have essentially become one. We know that many habits are closely linked like this.

For example, driving a car is not referred to as turning a steering wheel and stepping on the gas and brakes. These habits are so tightly woven that they are now considered part of the same action that is called driving.

With food, the same caveat holds true and in general, the closer the linkage, the more difficult it is to break them apart. Thus, we have created some important changes with the place-of-eating technique. We have made food the center attraction, we have increased the awareness of the ingestion, we have supported the ingestion only in pleasant, comfortable settings. We have decreased the amount of eating by having fewer potential eating episodes, and so we have decreased total caloric intake. Food is now given a place "for itself" and for its sole enjoyment.

Physical Activity in Everyday Lifestyle

She was a middle-aged woman who never had trouble with weight control, yet she arrived in my office one afternoon, concerned that her twenty-pound weight gain over the last two years must be related to a "sluggish metabolism."

We discussed her lifestyle in depth. She had not moved, changed jobs, gotten married or divorced. Her home situation was stable, with two children grown up and in college. She exercised at the club three times a week for forty-five minutes on a bike and took aerobic workout classes. She denied vehemently a change in eating style or pattern. After a long discussion and a normal physical exam, we both decided to do in-depth food analysis records. She presented excellent food records the next week. Her intake was about fourteen hundred calories a day, with good variation and food choices. There were no obvious binges or gross maladaptive eating patterns.

Both of us, being a bit frustrated, decided to embark on behavior mod analysis, introducing a specific technique or task weekly. Slowing down, place of eating, records, and all the other techniques fell in line. Time continued to pass with little change in this patient's weight. She insisted on checking her metabolic rate, which we did and calculated her basal metabolic rate to be about twelve hundred calories. We decreased calories, but this became difficult for this patient. One day while discussing a food record with her, I again brought up the concept of lifestyle change. I insisted that some changes must have occurred and prodded her mind for any possibilities.

She thought it over and then out loud, mulling over the possibilities, blurted out, "There was an aunt who passed away. Jim fractured his arm in school, but this was minor, and then there was the passing of Fluffy."

"Who was Fluffy?" I asked. She was the patient's home dog that had literally grown up with the family. About two years ago, at age fourteen, she became ill and passed away. The patient vividly remembered the dog and how dear she was to her. "I couldn't replace Fluffy though my husband wanted another dog, I just couldn't."

There was silence in the room. My face lit up with a gleam. I asked excitedly, "Who walked the dog?" She admitted both she and her husband had. She walked her two times a day, he in the evening once a day. She walked approximately ten blocks each time. I exclaimed, "That's it." She seemed amazed. I whipped out my calculator and began counting, ten blocks two times a day equals twenty blocks, or one mile, seven days a week at 365 days per year equals 365 miles times amount of calories per mile divided by 3,600 calories per pound. That would be 10.14 pounds per year times two years or the patient's newly acquired 20 pounds. It was amazing.

The patient literally had gained the exact amount of weight based on the lack of this one routine activity. It seemed too simple to be true, but it was. The physical activity of routinely walking the dog had been burning up 10.14 pounds of weight per year. When this ceased and all else was the same, the patient proceeded to gain weight at the rate of ten pounds per year. After thoroughly going over this concept with my patient, she accepted the idea of another dog. She returned to her physical activity and everyday lifestyle routine. Over the years she has slowly lost weight and I learned several years later that she was actually down in weight 22 pounds, pretty much back to her normal baseline weight.

I relate this story to you for a number of reasons. One is naturally to encourage increased physical activity in everyday lifestyle, and I don't mean playing tennis or golf (these are leisure activities). I am talking of the things that we do routinely: going to work, going shopping, etc. The second reason is to show you just how subtle a change in physical activity can be and the "ripple" effect it has over time. Many experts in the field of obesity still believe that the major cause of obesity is not so much in the overeating as it is in the underactivity. But I think, more important is the behavioral linkage that lack of activity causes. When one is inactive, food intake becomes much more available, more social, and more apt to occur in frequency.

We look at the "couch potato syndrome" and see this analogy immediately. People have increased their TV watching enormously to now over four hours per day. Television has become America's favorite pastime. There are more channels available. Fancier receptor units abound, and now multimedia contraptions (for want of a better term) are rapidly capturing our attention. The only work that we have is to punch a number on a selector or pre-program the whole bit once each week. We have become totally inactive.

After all, we need to relax after a long day in the office where we pound hard at our computer terminals! This lack of activity has shown up in our adolescents. In one recent study, the average American child has increased weight by 5.5 pounds and the weight gain has been directly linked to television. Worse than this is the food linkage that TV causes. We are bombarded by food commercials, two-for-one coupon offers, and ads for food. We watch TV programs in which food abounds and everyone seems to be eating. We overwhelmingly become more prone to eating ourselves. After all, we are sitting in a relaxed chair and immobile. It is easy to see how food links up with TV. This very joining-up compounds the problem because eating food becomes part of the whole event, and we no longer eat out of hunger but out of habit. Thus, the tenet of this technique is: "Man has become a lazy creature due to mechanization." Everything is automatic. The less work involved in doing something, the better. If I can park my car close to the office and get the elevator right up, I can sleep a bit later in the morning. G-d forbid I have to walk some extra steps!

Man has always been enthralled with gadgets that save time, automatic can openers, computers that shut off and turn on the house lights, escalators, speedy elevators, and voice-activated lights are all part of our busy lives. To better understand how behavioral change helps the situation, we must compare ourselves to the man of 1903.

One hundred years ago, life was very different. There was little mechanization. Most of the country lived on the farm. People did not own cars. Electricity in the house was a rarity. A typical day would begin by waking up early in the morning. Chores needed to be done before working the farm. Water was pumped from a hand pump or drawn from a well. Water was needed for washing up, washing the clothes, and cooking. Wood was chopped to have for kindling the stove and for the hearth.

An "outhouse" for toileting was truly outside the house. The horse had to be hitched and fed as well as the other animals. There was much more manual labor throughout the day. But beyond this, the man of 1903 accepted this hard manual labor as normal and part of his typical day. This was a pattern and not questioned.

If I had a crystal ball to see a hundred years into the future, I might be amazed to find that warp speed has been achieved and that people are not only "beaming" themselves up to the Enterprise but all over the planet. I might say to myself, "Wow, what a timesaver this beamer is," but because none of this technology exists at present, I don't complain and say, "Why is this car taking so long to get through the traffic? I should have beamed myself there." Instead, this is an acceptable pattern of living.

A Down to Earth Technique

Getting back down to earth, we need to ask: What are the techniques that we can use now to increase physical activity in everyday lifestyle? Like most techniques, they will only work if they are positively supported. I would never in troduce a technique of climbing up fifty flights of stairs to my office instead of taking the elevator because even if I could do it on a daily basis, I would find it quite onerous and negatively supported since the annoyance of doing it would predominate. Now, suppose I committed myself to getting off the elevators just two floors below my destination and climbing two flights instead. Though at first the technique seems odd, it is doable and does not feel punishing. However, the positive support behind it is weak—the knowledge of burning some extra calo-ries. A better technique would involve one that supports more than just the weight loss.

For example, did you ever take a cab to a Broadway show? You can be trapped in traffic for one hour just to go two or three blocks. Getting out of the cab three or four blocks away from your destination not only burns calories and saves money, but it will get you there faster. This pattern is thus supported by three positive reinforcers. There are many techniques that will increase physical activity in everyday lifestyle, some more posi-tively supported than others. I will mention a few here.

Parking the car can save time if it is closer to your office, but you may find parking lots a lot cheaper two to three blocks farther away from the office. The positive reinforcer of burning some extra calories, plus saving money, outweighs the slight convenience of the car being closer. Still other features may fit in. The car attendant may be horrible at the garage close by, but right on target at the one two or three blocks away. Indeed, he may save you time by getting the car out quicker and safer. Obviously, you can see how complicated these techniques can get.

Walking is always a useful technique. What few people realize is that small amounts of walking, a few steps here and a few steps there, soon add up. For example, when our automatic television selector went bad, I had to get up to change the channels. I didn't feel that inconvenienced since I was getting in the extra activity of walking up and back to the set.

So you see, going up steps instead of the elevator, escalator, or taking buses, subways, or cabs two or three blocks away from your destination and walking the rest of the way can work well in burning off calories over long periods of time.

Your task therefore is to look at your everyday routine from waking up until bedtime, and with that time, try out one or two techniques that require you to use your own body's energy. Remember to positively reinforce the habit and remember that it can be even a short, simple task. Over time the dividends will pay off and be substantial.

VISUAL CUES: THE ABCS OF STIMULUS CONTROL

When one thinks of behavior mod, one thinks of the classic "Pavlovian theory" with the dog, the bell, and the food. Or perhaps the more recent "Skinner" experiments with rats running through mazes for a snack.

In this section I will discuss the core techniques that

were originally developed in behavior modification to control eating habits. Control of eating behavior in its essence means to address the issues behind the habit. That is, what are the stimuli or antecedents a: that induce the eating behavior b: or for that matter turn off the habit? Finally, what are the consequences c: that occur after a behavior is enacted? Very simply put, the above are called the "ABCs" of eating behavior. In its simplest form, an ingestion of food has one "A" stimulus (food), one "B" behavior (eating it), and one "C" consequence (the completion of the action).

But in most instances, an ingestion of even the simplest food is more complicated than that. There may be several stimuli: a: smell of cheesecake—it looks good and I'm in the mood. This leads to b: I will eat it, I'll chew it, I'll just buy it, and c: it was delicious, I feel guilty about eating it, I threw it away, or I'm no longer hungry.

All of the above choices or combination of choices are possible. Behavior modification seeks to readjust habit by altering the initiators, responses, and consequences so that in the long run, one either eats less in calories or increases activity more. The result is a resetting of patterns that give us the end results that we want to see, which are weight loss and weight maintenance.

When a bunch of habits get linked together either by practice or by chance, a behavioral chain of events is formed. Each link in the chain is either one or multiple ABCs and each link can be supported or broken. It is the ability to manipulate the chain that defines the very essence of behavior modification. To make this clearer, let me define a situation with two different outcomes.

The first outcome is an original pattern that causes one to

eat and gain weight. The second outcome in the chain causes the same person to not eat and to lose weight. We look at the following scenario: Initiator one—Argument at work leads to Initiator two—passing a gourmet grocery like Zabar's in New York, leading to Initiator three—buying two cheese salami heroes. The next Initiator is going home angry, followed by still another link in the chain, sitting down alone in a chair and watching TV. The next link in the event is watching a boring TV program. The following link—going to the refrigerator, grabbing a giant hero, and eating it. The next link—after eating, an upset feeling of guilt and the following link—going back to eat the remaining hero.

The Need for Blockades

Now, let's look at this entire chain of events with a bunch of behavioral blockades that can occur anywhere along this chain. Here the patient has practiced possible behavior breakage events. The initial argument at work could have been subdued by talking back to one's boss and explaining the situation, perhaps even getting a bonus and turning the whole thing around. This would cause the lack of an urge to eat and the patient would be home free.

How about passing Zabar's? A second break in the chain could occur there. Purposely rewarding oneself by going past another store and looking for some other reward like a new set of jewelry or a pair of shoes, or something non-food that is considered a treat. One now feels better about oneself, and there is no urge to eat.

The next event was buying the actual food. Suppose this person makes the smarter choice in the store and buys fruit instead. This again would break the chain. Notice that the chain is getting closer to the final event of ingestion. Instead of the patient going home angry, he could have gone and had a massage at a spa or perhaps gone to the health club to relax and loosen up.

Finally, instead of sitting down in a chair and watching TV, the patient could have gone to his friend's house to talk about things and feel better about the day's events. The patient could have shut off the boring TV program and instead gotten involved with an exciting "Star Wars" computer game. Instead of going to the refrigerator and picking up the hero sandwich, the patient could have taken a walk outside or grabbed a different item, such as fruit. Eating the hero is already closing in on the last number of chain events. But still, even here, if the patient had second thoughts and ultimately decided that the ingestion would be a sabotage, he could have thrown away the hero after two bites.

At the onset of feeling upset about eating, he could have felt better tossing out the rest of the sandwich. Finally, eating the second hero as a punishment for guilt, the patient could have rethought the whole situation. Again, throwing away the second hero and deciding to start tomorrow with a "clean slate."

The above two scenarios show how a chain of events can be broken at each step using behaviorally learned techniques. Obviously, the earlier the chain is broken, the safer the individual is from having an anger-induced ingestion. Still, even late in the chain, breaks are very useful in restructuring one's thinking about oneself, gaining confidence, and redeveloping patterns that will be less destructive in the end. With this initiative in mind, we are ready to start learning about stimulus control.

STIMULUS CONTROL—THE STRICT AVOIDANCE TECHNIQUE

An old adage quoted from Confucius and many other behaviorists is: "Out of sight, out of mind" . . . or in our case, "out of mouth!" As simple as it seems, when food is not readily available, it is not eaten. From the extremes of being lost in the wilderness without food or water to forgetting to go shopping on the weekend, when food is not in sight, the stimulus to eat it is clearly diminished. This technique is relatively simple but very powerful.

Let's begin with simple examples. I leave my office to go downtown. If I take First Avenue, I pass the "deadly candy store," though most of the time I will not enter. There is the occasional yen for fudge that lights up my mind when I smell the aroma and see the freshly made fudge in the window. Perhaps one in five times passing, I go in for just one piece of fudge and then continue on my way. Now, let's suppose I purposely go another route, York Avenue, or whatever street that is quiet and tree-lined. I do not pass the store, and the image of fudge remains obliterated in my subconscious. I have saved myself 300 calories or so and never realize the desire for fudge. Though this technique appears absurdly simple, it works.

Advertisers on television know this technique very well. That's why you are bombarded with TV food commercials, showing you delectable foods, juicy, scrumptious and colorful. The advertisers know that if the idea is put in your mind via visual cues, you may just go out and get it. So here is another danger to watching TV. The strict-avoidance technique in this case would be to watch public TV or a video, strictly avoid the commercials, or not watch television at all.

Strict-avoidance techniques are also important at the office while you are at work. We all know about the proverbial "coffee break." So much of the time, there are cakes, snacks, and other items right next to the coffee. We don't intentionally look for them, but once in sight, we say, "Why not?" or "Boy, I haven't had this colorful type of doughnut for months." In each instance it is the visual cue that sets us off. We can avoid the snack by always keeping the coffee alone in a separate area or, if necessary, have someone else get the coffee for you.

How about celebrations? Here it is more difficult. Food is served in a beautiful fashion, and everybody is in a celebrating mood. But once again, by not looking around and staying out of harm's way, one is able to avoid hors d'oeuvres, etc. This is provided you did not pre-plan to have this food to begin with. I will talk about pre-planning as a technique in the next section.

Shopping and Storing Technique

One of the most powerful strict-avoidance techniques is "shopping and storing technique" that is done right at home. The home is a very dangerous place when it comes to eating. This is because of the ready availability of food there. All one has to do is to go to the refrigerator or cupboard and grab a favorite food. Worse than that, many homes are literally "set-ups" for eating.

I remember visiting a friend's home when I was a little kid. Every room had food in it. The living room had a piano, a television set, and three to four beautiful little dishes loaded with Hershey's kisses, M&M's, and nuts. The kitchen had a giant cookie jar filled with chocolate chip cookies and Oreos, probably two to three boxes worth. In my friend's bedroom were numerous candy bars spread out on his desk, as one would line up a group of prize trophies. It was as if you could not help but eat something when you were in that home. Of course, as a kid, I loved it, but when one is worried about trying to lose weight, this house was like a "wired time bomb." Strict-avoidance technique in the house starts with the food that we bring into the home.

Generally, we shop in large food stores that have a dozen or more brands of just about any food. In fact, the food stores are set up to induce us to buy things based on visual and taste cues. I walk into my local supermarket and ask for the produce section. It is way in the back of the store. To get to it, I might pass two aisles of "junk foods" ten feet high. These foods are in colorful eye-level packages, and indeed many of these foods can be seen right through their clear cellophane packaging. They almost call out to you to buy them.

Right next to the produce section is a fresh bakery section. There are two to three workers offering you a taste of the latest sensation—raspberry cheese cake with lemon fluff topping. They come up to you with a smile saying, "Just try this; it's our special of the day!"

You are persistently bombarded with these visual cues. Even on the cashier's waiting line, huge rows of junk candy and gum are conveniently lined up, hoping to be chosen by perhaps you or your child who is bored waiting in line.

This is no accident. Supermarkets are there to sell you food, and the owners and marketing people know very well how powerful visual cues are. Well, how does one combat this? Probably the most powerful technique is to make a pre-planned shopping list before you go, but make sure you have already eaten and are not hungry before creating the list. This ensures us of thinking rationally about what to shop for.

Try grouping the food based on your knowledge of where this food is located in the store. List all canned foods together, then paper goods, then frozen foods, etc. Try to plan the list to get around the "danger" parts of the store.

Next, shop for foods that are appropriately pre-packaged for you. For example, if you must buy cheese, you are better off getting the pre-sliced individually wrapped slices rather than buying a huge cube of cheese, which, when you are hungry, yearns to be eaten in large chunks. Even buying such foods as cereal in individually portioned boxes, though more expensive, will help to keep you focused when it comes to portion size.

When you are ready to shop, make sure you have already had a meal so that hunger does not sabotage you when you are in the supermarket. Inside the market, have all the items you have bought bagged conveniently for expeditious storage when you get home. Once home, store all food right away. Don't leave things conveniently around the table or on the counter. Storage is a crucial technique.

Out of Sight, Out of Mind

Store all foods out of sight. If you have to have dangerous foods, like cheese or high-fat items, in the home, place them way in the back of the refrigerator out of sight. Put the healthy foods in the front of the refrigerator in clear plastic bags for fruits and veggies. Store the danger foods in aluminum foil in the back of the refrigerator where they are less noticed.

I remember once going into my refrigerator in search of "risky food." I just had a yen for some Swiss cheese and remembered buying some a while back. I looked in the refrigerator and easily found the fruit up front. I rummaged through the back, opening up some tinfoil, which revealed a stored onion.

Then I found a stale half-apple in another tin. I was about to give up the search when I opened a third aluminum- wrapped item. It was the cheese all right, but uh-oh, it was all moldy. Basically then, my storage technique was successful.

The hidden cheese had gone unnoticed for a couple of weeks and fortunately for me had gone bad. The harder it is to get to a particular food, the less likely one is to eat it on the spur of the moment. Thus, cookies way up in the closet in individual packages out of sight are less likely to be nibbled on than cookies staring right out at you from the notorious cookie jar.

The Food Inventory

When it comes to food storage in the house, one of the smartest things to do is to do a food inventory list. Look throughout the house and decide whether or not you really need to have certain foods around. Many of my patients can use excuses to keep certain food in the house: "You never know when company will drop in," "How can I have an empty pantry when so-and-so drops by." The trouble is so-and-so only drops by once or twice a year, but the food is stored there in preparation daily. This is clearly a sabotage to the strict avoidance and pre-planning technique, and so these readily available foods tend to thwart us 365 days a year.

Another classic sabotage is the "I am in a rush, so let's order in" or, "Pick up that KFC on the way home." This usually is the route of least resistance, but, like any other habit, when repeated enough, it becomes part of one's lifestyle. Behaviorally, the answer to the problem is again strict avoidance and pre-planning. Have healthy pre-planned foods in the house if you are tired, in a rush, and have no time. Have healthy frozen dinners in reserve in the freezer. Many of them, like Healthy

Choice or Weight Watcher's, are well balanced, low in fat, and well portioned out.

Why waste precious calories when you are tired and rushed? It is best to reserve these precious calories for a time when you will be well rested and relaxed so that you can truly enjoy the meal. Thus, the positive reinforcer of eating a small, boring, frozen dinner is cognitive in nature. You have to feel that you are not truly going to enjoy a high-fat, quick fix when you are tired and rushed and that you would only be wasting calories at this point. But you kind of know that you would probably like to eat out on Saturday night after this grueling work week is over. This type of pre-planned motivation makes it well worth the switch, and you still feel you have earned something in the end.

Take It to the Bank

The strict-avoidance technique works well in and of itself but has much of its power enhanced by a technique called pre-planning and banking. This technique is a visual cue technique. Much of the time, our cue to eat is based on the time of day. One o'clock—time for lunch; six P.M.—time for dinner, or is it that we have been conditioned to eat because of the time of the day, not because of hunger.

How many times has a colleague at work said, "I'm going out to the x-y-z deli. Can I pick you up a ham and cheese sandwich?" You say, "Why not?" But the reason "why not" is because you're really not hungry yet! Therefore, we see many different types of initiators as a stimulus for us to eat. Much of the time, the only true indicator to eat—hunger—is left out.

Now, how does one get control? The answer is to pre-plan the meal or meals beforehand. Many of us do this for certain meals, such as packing the lunch box the night before to prepare for lunch the next day. This pre-planning ensures us of the certainty of that ingestion.

Before going to my office, I pack a bunch of fruit the night before, and as long as I remember to grab the brown paper bag, I am ensured of my boring but healthy lunch the next day. Pre-planning does create certainty. Once the food is on my credenza in the office, it becomes the pathway of least resistance. It is easy to grab a piece of fruit between patients. It is convenient. The desire for other food is diminished because in a sense my pre-planning has also supported a strict-avoidance technique. I have no need to go out to search for food or to pass other stores. I am only occasionally sabotaged when someone inadvertently brings in a "danger food," like a bagel or doughnut.

Now, some of you will say that pre-planning and strict avoidance lead to boring, non-spontaneous choices and ingestions, and in a sense this is true. But remember that it is the very boredom and control that diminish the stimulus to overeat food. The fewer choices and visual cues to eat, the less one eats. Probably the most classic example of this to the dieter is the "liquid formula diet," which has been around for decades.

A liquid formula diet is a well-balanced liquid protein drink, which is to be taken three or four times a day. Nothing else is eaten. Many patients tell me how they are never hungry despite being on only 800 to 1,200 calories each day. The decrease in hunger occurs for several reasons. There is in the strictest sense complete stimulus control and pre-planning. The patient knows what he will be eating for the next several weeks or months. There is marked diminishment in choice, generally chocolate or vanilla flavor, and that's it. So strict avoidance is at its fullest. Indeed, most patients do well on formula if they are not bombarded by other visual cues, such as sabotaging the diet with solid foods or suddenly going to an unplanned party, etc.

Numerous experiments have proven the validity of the above technique. We know that when rats are given healthy "rat chow," they stay nice and lean. If you give them "junk food," candy, cake and popcorn, they overeat and become obese. Human studies also show validity to the above. When patients are placed in a room with just formula to eat and no other food stimulus is available, the obese patients all lose weight till they approach a normal weight while the lean patients maintain their normal weight. These types of experiments done in the 1950s and 1960s led to the development of our classic behavioral techniques. It explains why the simpler a meal is, the less of it that is eaten.

Well, all this sounds great and dandy, except for one major problem: Most of us rapidly get bored. We lose weight and then get tired of the diet. We become easily sabotaged by outside forces. What generally happens is that we accept the first two Rs of the behavior mod, "Realization and Regimentation," but we cannot accept the third R, "Reorientation" to this eating style on a permanent basis. After all, how many people can live on formula for the rest of their lives or for that matter, fruit? Very few indeed.

What I am saying here is that despite being positively reinforced initially, there is just not enough positive reinforcement for most of us to continue these diets for a long period of time. For most of us, variety is truly the "spice of life." The above explains why most diets that are very monotonous fail. The reorientation is never there. People don't defend their weight loss and yo-yo back up. Behaviorally, we have an answer to this.

It is called "Banking and Shifting Calories." It is a critical part of Reorientation.

The third R requires the patient to fully accept techniques that not only create weight loss but ultimately protect the weight from returning. Many of us are willing to practice harsh restrictions to lose the weight; seeing those pounds come off is enough of a reinforcer to continue those tough diets.

But what happens when you've lost the weight and are just maintaining weight with the scale staying the same while there is a desire to still lose another ten pounds? That's when we usually get upset with the diet and feel like failures. The positive reinforcement is weak, and there is a vulnerability to easily break off from the diet. Thus, one must employ a positive reinforcement to sustain a habit continuously. Enter the "Banking" technique.

A Bank Paying Good Dividends

In banking and shifting calories, we are able to create a scenario that will be tolerable and even positively reinforced. The concept of banking is an easy one. Say we pre-plan out a meal that is basically healthy and monotonous at about 1,200 calories per day. And let's further suppose that at 1,800 calories a day, our weight stays the same and at 1,500 calories, we lose about one and a half pounds a week in weight. Now comes the fun part.

We can successfully pre-plan to have 1,200 calories per day for five days and bank 300 calories per day, or 1,500 calories per weekly total. This surplus of 1,500 calories can now be expended on the weekend, let's say for a nice Sunday meal out at a restaurant. We can now spend a total of our base 1,200 calories, plus the 1,500 additional, for as much as 2,700 calories.

With this situation, the individual in our case would still lose one and a half pounds in weight over the week and at the same time have a variety of food in his lifestyle.

In my practice, I find most patients need to have the "elasticity" to bend and shift calories in this fashion. Thus, pre-planning and banking together can in a very controlled way earn us the freedom most dieters yearn for. Through pre-planned control, one literally gets an increased sense of freedom to eat those truly enjoyable meals that we all look forward to. By having the ability to do this, several tenets follow: (1) Our diet is more positively supported and seems more realistic and doable; (2) We have the ability to look forward to special occasions and meals without the usual guilt attached when eating is uncontrolled; and (3) The monotony of 100 percent continuous dieting is broken. We no longer have to feel that a diet is 100 percent or no diet at all. We literally start to learn the "gray zone" in dieting. This concept of the "gray zone" is so important that an entire chapter is going to be spent analyzing it later on in the book.

Several precautions about banking calories—generally you can bank calories for up to two to three weeks, so don't start banking for Christmas parties in August or all you will be doing is resetting your "calorie goal" lower for several months and then yo-yoing back up in December. Banking calories should have a specific purpose or occasion in mind, although many of my patients bank some calories for the weekend even if they are not sure what is coming up. Never take a "credit line" on banking calories. That is, never overeat and then say, "I'll just decrease eating all of the next week."

Like a real credit line, one feels less secure in this situation, perhaps even more guilty about everything and, in a way, just like a credit line punishes you with credit interest payments, so also paying back calories has a punishing-like quality to it. It is much safer and better to feel "I have money in the bank to spend."

Finally, if you do spend calories saved, don't overspend. Budget these calories and get back to your original eating-style pattern the very next day. I have had several patients bank calories for the weekend and then get sabotaged by continuing their high-calorie eating style into the next week. You must be able to make a sharp clean cut after the meal and get right back on track with your original style. This is called "shaping the behavior." Many patients fear this technique because they fear they might lose control once they start eating the banked calories. However, with guided practice and cautious accurate food records, most of these patients get over the fear of loss of control.

Visual Cues: European-Style Serving

If you're Amish, celebrate Thanksgiving, or go to a Chinese restaurant—you have at one time or other eaten "American Style." This type of eating is when food is served on platters and brought to the table. The platters are passed around, and everyone takes what they want. If we are still in the mood, we go for seconds. The problem with this is from a visual cue standpoint, we are encouraged to eat more. The food is plentiful and right in our sight. It smells good, tastes good, and other people at the table are taking seconds, all cues stimulating us to have more. In other words, the path of least resistance is to eat.

Behaviorally, the answer to this is "European-Style

Serving." The term comes from observing the service at some of the most prominent European restaurants. In this scenario, food is served in individual plates brought to the table separately. You know, when the silver cover is over the plate, your waiter announces, "Dinner is served!" and he whips off the cover. Even dinner rolls are served separately. Behaviorally we eat what is in front of us, but this time around, portion is automatically controlled and unless we are "big spenders," second portions don't occur. In a sense, the "out of sight, out of mouth" concept occurs. This technique should be brought to your home.

To do this may take a little more work but should not take away from the enjoyment of eating. Food can be prepared in the correct portion size or, if there is a family involved, the food can be portioned out in the kitchen and brought out by another person who is in control of the kitchen. Baskets of rolls or platters are strictly taboo. Most patients will get used to this technique quickly, and it usually will save calories over the long run. A point about portion control here: large food companies like Heinz, Weight Watcher's, and Diet Centers have made a billion-dollar industry out of pre-portioned, pre-planned frozen dinner meals. They know those meals are balanced and automatically portioned out.

Let's look at two scenarios: the family is rushed in both situations. In one, the family desires to get some "fast food" on the way back from work: Chinese food, pizza, fried chicken, or whatever. The family members are tired and hungry. They open the food on the table and go for it. There is no portion control. The food is generally high in fat and oils. In some situations, like pizza, the food is eaten right out of the box and not even put on plates. There is a total lack of awareness in quality and quantity of food eaten, and food is generally overeaten.

In the second scenario, the family has a variety of frozen dinners stocked in the freezer. They also have fruit and fresh vegetables in the refrigerator. They too come home, tired and rushed. The frozen dinners are "nuked" in the microwave and the vegetables, salad, and fruit are ready to eat. The meals are automatically portioned out. Only the salad and fruit can be overeaten to any extent. This family has saved their precious time but has eaten with much better portion control, has had dramatically less fat and oil in their meal, and finally, has a much greater awareness of what they ate. This family has not overeaten.

Plate and Utensil Size

Though these techniques seem obvious, they are perhaps the most seldom used. That's because we humans tend to be lazy creatures of habit. For example, I use a large plate to eat because I don't want to get up again and I can fit more in a large plate. I use large utensils because I can get to my food more conveniently with fewer mouthfuls. Behaviorally, we want to change these habits because both of the above are more conducive to overeating.

Did you ever run out of large plates and were too lazy to wash them? You grab one of those smaller salad plates and put your macaroni and cheese onto it. You really were short of space and tried to heap it up even on this smaller plate but still ended up with a portion size smaller than usual. I remember once being in a restaurant. I had finished my appetizer using a shrimp cocktail fork. The main dish came, but the usual size fork was missing. I started to eat my baked potato with the small fork. Boy, it seemed like it took forever to eat the food and it actually seemed like I was eating more.

These techniques are visual cues. When you put the same amount of food in a plate that is smaller than usual, the portion size looks humongous. When you take a biteful of food with a small fork, it appears as if you have eaten even a greater amount of food. The reality is that you will almost always end up eating less.

Practicing these techniques at home is relatively easy. Just put those big dinner plates in storage and make them hard to get to. Now you stick with just salad-sized plates and you will see over time a diminution in overall portion size. Plate-size technique in a way mimics the "frozen dinner technique." Look at the size of a "Healthy Choice" or "Weight Watcher" meal. It is quite small. Some of these meals come complete with dessert and topping, but if you paid close attention to them, they are dramatically restricted in size. It is for this reason that these meals are weight-reducing.

In another plate-size technique, you can try playing some nutritional games with the plate you eat from. Most of us serve the main dish of food, which is usually high in calories in a regular-size plate and put the side dish, usually a healthy vegetable or salad in one of those small round dishes. Now try reversing what you eat. Put the fish, chicken, or meat in the small dish and place the vegetable or salad on the larger plate. The net effect is that you have become more nutritious in your eating and you are taking in less calories.

Empty Plate Syndrome

One of the most difficult visual cues that I have come across is the "Empty Plate Syndrome." This technique involves the ability to leave some food over on the plate and not devour the whole portion. This technique is important because what it basically seeks to accomplish is to separate out eating food for reasons of hunger from eating food because it is in front of you or because you have been "conditioned" to finish everything on the plate.

Do you remember being at the dinner table when you were growing up. Maybe you were not really hungry on certain occasions. You wanted to go out and play, but your parents insisted, "Eat everything on that plate or go to your room." You tried spreading the food out over the plate to make it look as if you had eaten, but it never seemed to work. Then your parents might have made you feel guilty, "how can you leave that food, just think about those poor, starving children in Ethiopia" (depending on when you grew up, the country changed; Europe was in the WWII era, the early 1950s for the Korean War, the '60s for Vietnam, Biafra, etc.). Boy, did we "starve" a lot of people by not finishing everything on our plate. Or at least that's how our parents made us feel. Now you might say, I am a rational grown-up today.

But these talks at the table have been continuously brainwashed into us. We take a bowl of soup and sip it down to the last teaspoon. We take a piece of bread to wipe the plate clean. We do this even though our body cues tell us we are full.

To break these patterns, we must practice leaving a bit of food left over on the plate. This takes conscious practice and constant awareness of one's true hunger. It also takes rationalizing the fact that you will not be punished and should not feel guilty in wasting food. After all, the food you leave over has no effect upon whether the people across the ocean starve or eat. You might find it easier to just leave a small morsel of food behind so that you have a sense that something is left over. Ultimately, if you get used to leaving something on your plate, you will go more by your true hunger cues and less by your emotional or visual cues.

Restaurant Eating

One of the biggest problems I face with my patients is the patient who is the frequent "restaurant eater." Whether because of business or entertainment, many patients will eat out four or more times per week. Part of the problem at the start is to convince these patients that (1) this frequency of eating out is too much, (2) when you eat out a lot, you must consider the restaurant as if it were your home and plan meals accordingly, and (3) generally, meals served in restaurants are not dieter friendly.

Most restaurants serve too much food, and good nutrition is frequently lacking. First on the list is to ask whether you truly have to eat out this frequently. You may be eating out to socialize, and there may be many alternate activities that would still permit you to socialize without food being intricately involved. Even with business and entertainment, alternate activities can get you away from the three-martini lunch. Take your client out to the golf course or to a show on Broadway. Then go to a café for some cappuccino. I will discuss the powerful technique of alternate activities in another chapter.

Once you realize that you are doomed to eat out frequently despite alternate activities, you must reshape your attitude towards the restaurant. The restaurant must be looked at as most of us look at our kitchens. Many of my patients have a restaurant quota of one to two eat-outs per week. The rest of the time is spent eating healthy and saving calories for these one or two restaurant meals.

What I tell the frequent restaurant goer to do is to ask which one to two meals out are really important to them. Then to look at the other meals as being healthy "at home type meals." This requires a number of techniques including the all-important pre-planning technique. It also involves using the techniques just mentioned in this chapter. Pre-planning is ultimately the most important because it addresses the behavioral link early on. If you pre-plan to eat out at a salad bar, you will have avoided difficulties to begin with. Pre-planning the restaurant that one will go to is just the start. You should also pre-plan the type of meal that you will have there. In other words, don't wait until you get to the menu to decide what you will eat. Decide early on.

The menu itself can be a big sabotage, especially if there is a delectable list of specials. Most people who eat out frequent the same restaurants all the time. They know the basic menus. You can avoid getting sabotaged if you carefully plan the meal beforehand. In fact, many restaurants get to know you so well that they go out of their way to cater to your needs.

This may include serving you that broiled fish without the sauce, but they may also prepare foods specifically for your needs. In one case, the restaurant owner prepared the shrimp cocktail as a main dish with additional shrimp, though this was not particularly on the menu. In another case, the restaurant owner knew not to serve bread at the table. Obviously these restaurants want you back and will go out of their way to please you, so take advantage of this. The more pre-planned you are beforehand, the less likely you are to get sabotaged or surprised by unexpected specials or only having foods that are fattening on the menu. This technique alone will save you numerous calories.

The next thing you want to do is to ask yourself which one or two meals would be your real eat-out meals and which should be pre-planned more as diet meals. Pre-planning the diet meal can take advantage of some of the techniques that we just spoke about.

Go to a restaurant that serves European-style and avoid the bulky American-style restaurant. To control portion size, take advantage of the appetizer portion size served in many restaurants. You can control portion and plate size if you ask that your main dish be the appetizer portion of that specialty. I knew a patient who would go to his favorite Italian restaurant. He was well pre-planned. He would start the meal by asking the waiter to bring fresh celery and carrots on ice. The bread was not brought to the table (the waiter knew not to bring it). He would then have a fresh salad, and for the main dish, he had the appetizer-size portion of pasta in light tomato sauce. For dessert he had a fresh bowl of strawberries. This meal was dramatically decreased in calories when compared to the main menu.

Other restaurant techniques involve having Balsamic vinegar on salad, not the heavy caloric dressing that most restaurants serve. Also, as a general rule, avoid any foods with sauce since they generally contain hidden calories in the form of oil. Another interesting technique is the one-half portion idea. This is a carryover from the one-half sandwich and cup of soup for lunch pattern that many restaurants have adopted. Several of my patients automatically have one-half their main dish saved for another night or they share the main dish with a friend. Whatever they decide to order for the main dish, it is automatically cut in half.

Clearly, you can once again see the familiar trend. The earlier in the chain of events you are careful and pre-plan, the less likely you are to get into trouble. Though the one-half meal is a great pattern, it is late in the behavioral chain. In other words, you risk eating the whole portion since you are one step away from saying to the waiter, "I'll have a steak" instead of "Please cut the steak in one-half for my friend and me."

VII

NUTRITIONAL TECHNIQUES

THERE are many nutritional books and gurus out there today. Most of these techniques are based on strict nutritional changes and ignore other behavioral techniques. Many of these techniques are not nutritionally sound or compromise the nutritional health of the individual.

My goal in the next three chapters is to put forth a behavioral lifestyle that is nutritionally sound and meets the minimum ADA requirements. I will also show you how to use nutrition as a technique in itself. When I was in med school, there were no nutritional courses and I was ignorant of sound nutritional techniques. I learned most of my nutrition by taking a Specialty Fellowship in Endocrinology, Metabolism, and Nutrition, and therefore I am writing this chapter simply, as if you were like me back in med school with little knowledge of good nutrition. These rules were developed to help patients make food decisions easily and on the spur of the moment:

Three Cardinal Rules of Nutrition

Rule #1. "If you must eat animal products, the lighter

97

the color, the better." White chicken meat is healthier than dark. Veal is healthier than steak, the egg white healthier than the egg yolk.

Rule #2. "If you eat vegetable products, have it unrefined; if you eat animal products, refine it." So, in the vegetable arena, corn is better than its refined counterpart, corn oil. The whole apple is better than its refined product, apple juice. Whole wheat, high-grain bread is better than refined white bread. In the animal arena, just the opposite is true. Refined lean beef burger is better than the fatty natural burger. No sugar, no-fat yogurt is better than whole natural yogurt.

And the final cardinal rule:

Rule #3. "Always choose vegetable products over animal products." In general, vegetable product foods (from the ground) are much lower in fat and calories and devoid of cholesterol. They also offer the advantage of giving you more vitamins/minerals and nutrients as compared to animal products. Therefore, salad, steamed vegetables, or baked potato are better than steak, chicken, or fish. To ensure you I am not just encouraging you to become a macrobiotic freak (although from a health standpoint this is not necessarily a bad move), later on, I will introduce you to a method of enforcing these rules with various intensities.

The above three rules help you decide the healthier meal when given a choice. As usual, there are a few exceptions to the rule: olives, nuts, avocado and palm, though vegetable products, contain a lot of fat and therefore must be eaten cautiously and with portion control. What still must be learned is how to truly identify the food product eaten. In the next section, I will discuss the all-dangerous hidden calorie.

Beware the Hidden Calorie

One day I went with a friend to a Chinese restaurant. I had banked about 2,000 extra calories during the previous week and decided to "spend it" on a fried egg roll, ribs, and a sautéed fried chicken dish.

My friend was appalled at what I ordered and said, "How can a nutritionist order this? I am getting the boiled wonton soup, sautéed broccoli and eggplant and vegetable chicken in Peking sauce." At this point, I explained to my friend the danger of the hidden calorie. I was all upfront concerning my order. I told him I had banked calories all week for this particular meal. Indeed I had fruit for breakfast and lunch, four to five days before, and only healthy portion dinners. I had deposited 2,000 calories in the bank, and I was splurging on a very high-fat meal. But what I told my friend after this totally surprised him.

I told him that he was probably having as many fat calories as I was. I began to explain. The wonton with the pork inside had increased fat and the soup was not a broth but had high-fat content with oil floating on top. As for the broccoli and eggplant, it looked great and tasted great, but it was saturated with sesame oil. In fact, because of the increased surface area of the broccoli, there was probably an inordinate amount of oil soaked into the dish.

As for the vegetable chicken in Peking sauce, again it looked great, but the dish was saturated in a hot oil sauce. My friend was amazed. He said, "It looked so healthy with all those vegetables!" There was a bit of silence. I then ordered pistachio ice cream for dessert, and he watched me eat it. I have to admit I only eat this type of meal once every couple of months or so, but I tell you this story to demonstrate the difficulty many patients have with discerning the true caloric content of a food.

The situation is much worse than it seems because many manufacturers of food like to place healthy claims on their food products. We all see those boxes of cookies that say "100% fat free, no cholesterol," but a closer look reveals a high sucrose (sugar) content. Indeed, the cookies have nearly the number of calories as the old-fashioned counterparts. Unfortunately, food-labeling laws are deceiving, and companies take full advantage of them to make you think you are getting a healthier food.

Such claims as no fat per portion size can actually have some fat in the product but can be reported as no fat per ounce, etc. Other products are labeled "reduced fat" or "no choles-terol." For example, some cheeses say 50 percent less fat on the label, but this is 50 percent less fat by weight and not by calorie, so that the cheese that originally had 80 percent fat may be 55 to 60 percent fat, but the label may say 50 percent less! This type of gimmick is extremely common on many food items.

Use a Calculator

One must have a calculator and actually calculate total calo-ries for the entire product. Then divide it by the portion eaten. It sounds complicated, and it is. There are numerous proposed laws presently awaiting passage to reduce the confusion, but most food lobbies are against this passage. I therefore will now mention in my book a very useful manual of the food groups and their calorie contents: *Exchange Lists for Meal Planning*.

This book is supported by the ADA and the American

Dietetic Association. It is simple, precise, and most importantly teaches you how to calculate what's in a food.Other labeling gimmicks seen on food products include the words "all natural." This concept connotes a healthier food, but in reality foods that just don't have additives or are chemically man-made can pass under this guise.

For example, I was looking at a wafer bar that was labeled "made with natural fruit juice." On closer inspection of the label, I saw that the fruit juice was concentrated down, and the "natural sugars" from the juice were really the products put in the food. So the only difference between this food and a sugared food wafer was "who made the sugar?" Dow Chemical or the apple from Mother Nature? Molecule per molecule, these products have the same calories in sugar!

How about the concept of 100 percent? It is a nice round figure, but it too is used with a false premise. Think of products that say "This product is made from 100 percent all-natural fruit juice." Sounds good but we all know the sugar story from above and now, in addition, what else is the product made of? How about saturated coconut oil and palmitic oils or hydrogenated fats? Be careful concerning the words "reduced, or less than," etc. Reduced, compared to what or less than what?

In my practice I find that patients have difficulty discerning true caloric content of many foods because of the hidden calories. I have many patients who have changed their style of eating by using these products, only to find out that they have merely substituted different sugars or fats for their original meal. Patients also get carried away with the concept of "no fat or no cholesterol." They think they get a *carte blanche* on eating these items and don't realize that even healthier calories add up!

I had one patient who was thrilled with a zero fat, zero cholesterol frozen yogurt. He felt it was healthy. After all, yogurt itself connotes a healthy message of longevity—at least in Siberia—so why not eat frozen yogurt, especially if the fat is taken out? Unfortunately, this patient ate a full pint of frozen yogurt every night or approximately 600 calories worth of protein and sugar. Yes, there was no fat in the product, but there were calories and 600 of them to pop five nights a week. The patient gained forty pounds in only one year.

The upshot here is that all calories count. Portion control and prudent pre-planning will help avoid the above situation. As will simplifying what one eats. I am never worried that the apple, pear, or banana I had for breakfast had hidden calories. They have been produced the same, wholesome way for over one billion years. Now that's a track record!

THE ALL-VEGETABLE DAY TECHNIQUE

I have had so many patients in my practice tell me how they really tried to stay on a healthy diet. They were on Pritikin's Diet or the Dean Ornish Diet and actually did well for some time, only to falter down the road and go back to old, maladaptive nutritional patterns. Many patients meant well and do want to change. Unfortunately, they fail to perceive the enormous life-style change that this connotes. One problem here is people try to do something "all or none style," i.e., the light switch is either on or off. They unfortunately have difficulty learning about the "gray zone." Once again, it becomes much easier to make a lifestyle change piecemeal than to have a total upheaval. Patients ask often how to do this pattern change.

I describe to them an "all-vegetable day." The challenge here is to pick one day during the week where only products grown from the ground (vegetables, non-animal products) are consumed. Patients are asked to design nutritionally a day when breakfast, lunch, and dinner are all without animal by-products. For many patients this is an awareness technique that shows them nutritionally the quality of food. Many patients use this "all-vegetable day" as a banking day since it is generally low in calories. This one day is easy to handle since it is just one-seventh of what you can eat for the week. It can be positively supported because it serves as a health-awareness day from the strict nutritional standpoint, and it is an excellent technique for banking.

A Calorie Is a Calorie or Is It?

Many books, papers, and studies are written concerning the major differences in food types and their effect on health and weight. From the behavioral perspective, we note that patients can lose weight and maintain it by decreasing calories in general and increasing activity. But I feel obligated to tell you about food types because health and wellness are a big part of what behavioral change is all about. Indeed the type of food eaten—because of its quality— will either be weight and fat-promoting or weight and fat-demoting.

Let's look at several factors involved in the quality of food. One is caloric density. Caloric density is defined as the amount of calories consumed/over time equals caloric density. By strict definition, calorie-dense foods are foods high in fat and sugar and low in fiber and roughage and water, but we would like to broaden that definition to include total calories consumed over a certain period of time.

For example, a whole apple is low in calorie and in caloric density. You mechanically chew it and then swallow it which can take from ten to fifteen minutes. If we took the same apple and ground it into applesauce, it can be consumed in a few minutes. Note that the calorie content per portion size would be identical, but the caloric density of the applesauce would be far greater than the apple, thus the more ease in consuming the food, the higher the potential caloric density—even when caloric composition remains the same. Remember that the cardinal rule of nutrition states: "If it is vegetable, don't refine it." This is because even mechanical refinement can increase caloric intake, based upon the preceding rule.

Another quality of food is its ease of "digestion." By this, we mean the ability of food to be rapidly absorbed by the intestinal tract from the stomach. Though this index seems similar to our caloric density index, it really is not. Let's look at some examples.

First, in our above example, the apple and purée of apple, the apple is held up mechanically in the stomach till it is reduced to a semi-liquid. The applesauce requires much less work. Beyond the stomach, both food items are identical and absorbed at the same rate.

Now, let's look at ices on a popsicle versus the same liquid quantity of soda pop. The caloric density in each is quite different. The ice pop must be bitten into and eaten slower than the soda pop, so the soda pop has a higher caloric density. Once in the stomach, both these items are easily digested to simple sugars and readily absorbed. Thus, they are nearly identical in the ease of digestion. Note that calorically they are quite similar, containing almost totally simple sugars and water.

Finally, let's compare the solid ice pop to the apple purée. Caloric density is probably high for the purée, which is easily swallowed without being chewed or sucked. But the ease of digestion in this case is quite the opposite. The apple purée requires more enzymatic breakdown in the GI tract than the pure sugared liquid of the ice pop.

Thus, there is a decrease in the ease of digestion of the apple purée. Generally, foods with increased difficulty in digestion are higher in fiber. From the weight loss standpoint, the more difficult the digestibility of an item, the less one eats of it. Anyone who has had too many vegetables or fruit products know that at a certain level they will have increased gas, increased bowel movements, etc., since the ease of digestion is overwhelmed and the body can no longer handle the load. The patient becomes uncomfortable and stops eating at this point in time.

The Role of Insulin, Carbs, Fats, and Proteins

"The right fuel mixture for the right body." There is probably no pre-set diet that is correct for everyone. Just like engines, ideal fuel portion depends on engine type, performance, etc. The same is true in people. However, most overweight patients share one major metabolic feature in common—the production of insulin.

Insulin, as a hormone, is obeseogenic, that is insulin levels go up in the "fed state," and elevated insulin levels are associated with obesity. In fact, obese individuals as a whole are at high risk for developing diabetes mellitus because of increased insulin levels and a general resistance to the insulin effect. The more overweight one is, the higher the insulin level and resistance and the higher the risk for developing diabetes in one's lifetime.

On the contrary, the lean individual has low insulin levels, is highly sensitive to the Insulin effect, and has a much lower chance of developing diabetes. To complicate this situation, a whole host of negative metabolic factors go into effect when insulin levels are too high. This includes elevation of triglycerides (fat) in the body, elevated fat in the liver, elevated atherosclerosis formation, and the increased risk of hypertension, with increased risk of coronary artery disease and death. In essence, elevated insulin levels are linked to the classical diseases of Western Civilization, hypertension, heart disease, and sudden death. The corollary is that low insulin levels are a sign of health, leanness, and low risk for the aforementioned diseases.

Therefore, the diet designed for the obese, sedentary individual is one that helps diminish the insulin level in one's body. Of course, any weight loss in general will help decrease insulin levels, but specifically the culprits that we want to go after are the simple sugars and carbohydrates. These are foods that when digested turn into sugars, which of course stimulate more insulin to be secreted.

The ability to eliminate these foods will help decrease the insulin level. Now, separating these carbohydrates from the diet requires one to look at the entire spectrum of carbohydrates. We can easily tell you that sugar and refined wheat or pasta are insulinogenic, but in reality there is an entire spectrum with sugars on the worst end and carbohydrates and vegetables at the best end. Let's look at graph #1.

In the above situation, the more foods eaten toward the good healthy side, the less insulin generated and the healthier a person is. Remember again about the "gray zone." Don't try to be all or none with the above example.

A simple trend or shift towards the right is much more realistic than saying, "I'll just eat vegetables the rest of my life and nothing else." There are theoretical benefits of decreased insulin levels that have to do with appetite. There are theories that say increased insulin levels in the body correlates to increased insulin levels in the brain, and this is associated with increased hunger signals that emulate out from the brain. If this is true, insulinogenic foods are also foods that are less satisfying and tend to make you hungrier. The higher the insulin levels, the hungrier we get and the more we eat.

Graph #1

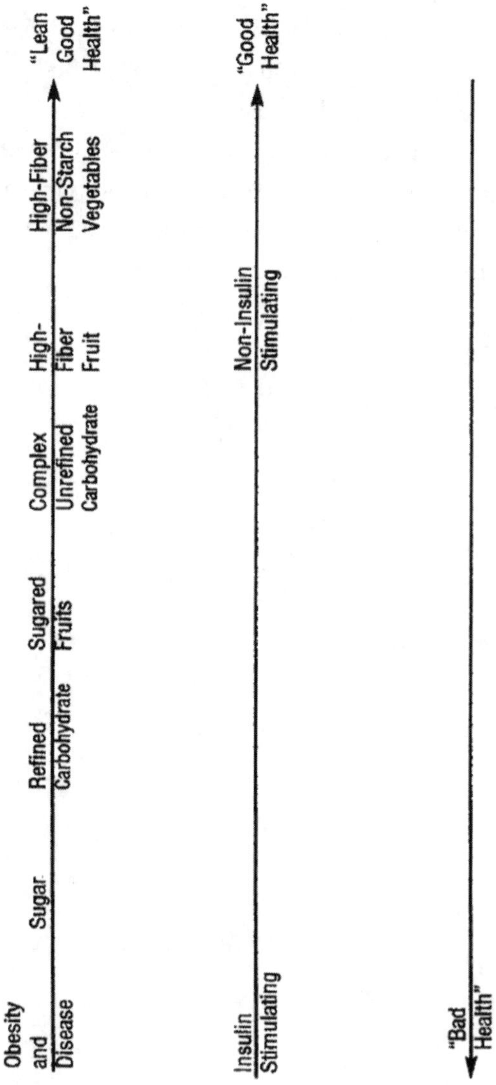

Sugar	Refined Carbohydrate	Sugared Fruits	Complex Unrefined Carbohydrate	High-Fiber Fruit	High-Fiber Non-Starch Vegetables

Obesity and Disease → "Lean Good Health"

Insulin Stimulating → Non-Insulin Stimulating → "Good Health"

"Bad Health"

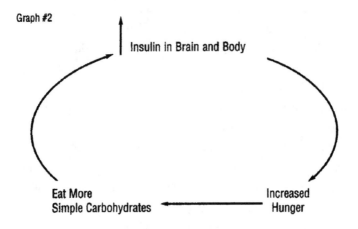

Graph #2

Many of my patients have described increased hunger and cravings especially after eating sweets or simple carbohydrates. Because of this, they have gained even more weight! When placed on a decreased carbohydrate, high-protein diet (Zonelike diet), they have successfully been able to lose weight with less hunger.

So now we know the diet for an obese individual should contain decreased simple carbohydrates. What about other food constituents? First, let's talk about fat. Traditionally through the 1980s, patients were told to eat 55 percent complex carbohydrates, 15 percent protein, and 30 percent fat. Though we have decreased the amount of simple carbohydrates, we still adhere to the concept of a low-fat diet. We would like to maintain a fat content in the diet at percent or slightly less. The lower the better, although recent literature now tells us that 26 percent is the ideal goal.

Fat is an essential nutrient and contributes to the taste of food. It is highly caloric. It has the highest calories per weight of food. Animal fats in particular contain saturated fat and cholesterol; however, even vegetable fats, such as those found in nuts, are caloric. Fat calories are also considered inert. Fat calories can be stored as fat gram per gram yielding approximately 100 percent caloric retention. Protein and carbohydrates need to be converted to fat and there is an energy-burning cost to do this. Thus, only about 77 percent worth of these calories end up stored as inert fat.

Now that we have reduced fat and simple carbohydrates, what about protein? Protein is the third essential nutrient. It has high nitrogen content and contains amino acids, the building blocks of muscle and cell constituent.

Protein comes from many sources: grains, beans, milk products, eggs, and animal sources (meat, chicken, fish, etc.). The quality of proteins are also different, with egg white considered a high quality source and the cartilage in meat a lower quality source. It is very important to note that one can satisfy one's protein needs from vegetable products (non-animal) alone. Protein is not insulinogenic. It is derived from lean animal sources, such as egg white, lean chicken, fish, and some lean meats. It is also tied into many vegetable products, beans, tofu, and oatmeal, to name a few.

Thus we can see that the ideal fuel mixture for the obese individual will contain low carbohydrate, low fat, and moderately high protein compared to past recommended diets. Remember that this Zonelike diet is the fuel for an obese individual who needs to lose weight.

Lean individuals, particularly those who are very aerobically active, have low insulin levels. They require elevated carbohydrate for energy production. They take excess carbohydrate and store it as muscle and liver "glycogen." These are starch deposits that permit the body to gain more energy on

an immediate basis. This becomes more important in competi-
tive sports where bursts of energy are critical. These patients
have low insulin levels and high glucagon levels, promoting the
formation of glycogen instead of inert fat.

For this reason, lean active individuals do better on a high-
carbohydrate, decreased-fat diet. Despite this factor they are
still better off not having simple sugars, as they are more prone
to a condition called reactive hypoglycemia in which even small
surges in insulin can cause a very low blood glucose.

What's the Story on Fiber?

Fiber is the inert, non-digestible portion of natural foods.
For the obese individual, fiber has two important features. One
feature is that fiber increases satiety, the feeling of fullness.
Since fiber is devoid of calories but has bulk, it fills up the
stomach reservoir. Increased stretching of the stomach wall
tells the brain via nerve networks to stop eating and thus one
feels full.

Many of my patients eat an increased fiber vegetable dish
before starting their regular meal. Examples of this are patients
loading up on celery, broccoli, carrots, etc. By the time the main
dish arrives, many of these patients have less hunger and end
up eating less of their caloric dish.

The fiber dish also serves as a "slowing down technique."
Since it mechanically takes time to chew these fiber dishes,
these patients automatically slow down the speed of eating and
feel less hungry. Fiber also serves another important function.
Both soluble and insoluble fibers are inert and serve as bulking
agents for the colon.

This is important for several reasons, including the fact that
patients need to have regular, comfortable bowel movements.

Constipation, diverticulosis, and colon cancer have all been associated with decreased fiber and elevated fat in diets. In countries where people eat very high-fiber diets, such as Africa, colon disease is virtually unheard of. The more Western the civilization, the less the fiber and the more the colon disease.

In our country, colo-rectal carcinoma is the second leading cancer-causing death. So much for fiber in the American diet. Soluble fibers also soak up water and help soften the bowel movement. Finally, fiber is important for the colon microcosm. For healthy bacteria to thrive and help digestion, they must get their share of fiber.

The Importance of Water

The human body is essentially made up of 60 percent water. Water is critical for nutritional transport and cellular survival. Consuming fresh water also serves other functions. It helps fill you up just like fiber does. Many patients consume many glasses of water or dietetic beverage before they start a meal to fill themselves up. Water also helps fiber do its job and thus helps in preventing colon disease.

Vitamins, Minerals and Micronutrients

Though the human body can essentially get its nutrients from food, most individuals have difficulty staying on a so-called "perfect nutritional diet." Patients who diet also tend to decrease their nutritional intake at least initially to lose weight. They decrease caloric intake overall and may therefore diminish intake of vitamins. Targeted foundation nutrition is a critical feature for maintaining overall optimal wellness and health.

In our discussion we will concentrate on nutritional support for the obese individual who is attempting to optimize wellness with weight loss. Several organ systems will be overtaxed when patients go on a reducing diet.

We will start with the upper gastrointestinal tract, as this is where food first enters the body. Patients on diets generally take in much less food. This creates an acid environment in the stomach. Since the acid is not buffered by food, patients may have increased peptic disease from overproduction of acid. These patients do well on natural acid buffers. In my practice, I use alkaline products. These products are natural with no side effects and effectively buffers and modulates acid products.

A smaller number of my patients are hypoacidic and require enzyme and hydrochloric acid. These patients will take a natural acidifying product for digestion.

From the stomach, we head toward the small bowel. This is the area of nutritional absorption. In patients on altered diets, which tend to have increased fiber, difficulty with digestive rates may occur. These patients develop bloatiness, gas, and occasionally abdominal pain. In this case I use another class of nutrition products called pancreatic enzymes. These products contain a natural, high-quality proteolitic lipase pancreatic enzyme mixture, which aids in the digestion and alleviates the acidic symptoms.

Food one eats now goes in two directions. One direction is fiber food to the colon. The second direction is absorbed food to the liver. Since we are in the GI system, let us look at the colon first. It is here where all the undigested fiber remnants end up. For patients on a diet, increased gas and abdominal pain may occur. These patients do well with high-quality fiber products in titrated doses. I use natural fiber with a good ratio of soluble to insoluble fiber. This aids in the intestinal elevation of water products.

The liver is the main warehouse where food is appropriately packaged and altered for its final destination—the human cell. Many things happen at the liver level. First, we have the nutrients coming in from the gut. These are the absorbable nutrients from the intestine that consist of amino acids, proteins, carbohydrates, and fat (triglycerides). Hopefully, if the patient is eating healthy, substances are stored in the correct ratio. Patients will require appropriate amounts of B and C vitamins to adequately metabolize nutrients. Many of my patients will use a ratio-balanced vitamin product, which has the appropriate B and C complex in it to ensure that they have the correct amount of these vitamins on hand.

However, a second very important thing is happening to the liver when one diets. The liver is being overwhelmed by huge amounts of fat released by the fat cells. Indeed this is why patients are losing weight. They are decreasing in the size of their fat cells. These cells are releasing fat as a nutrient because patients on a diet are in negative energy balance. That is because they eat less food than their body's energy requirements. The side reaction to the liver is that it can be overwhelmed by the amount of fat. It's like a Macy's sale, with everybody suddenly in line with just one cashier available! In this case, the liver requires nutrients to support fat metabolism.

In my patients I use natural products which contain choline. I also use Omega Fish Oils to support liver function. Liver micronutrients are carried by the blood stream to all the body's cellular sites. Here, these nutrients help build up cellular structure or are converted to energy for specific needs, such as cell production of muscular energy or pump function to initiate specific cellular function.

For example, kidney cells need energy to pump water out of the body. Brain cells need energy to initiate nerve impulses. Many of my patients will take specific vitamin products for their specific cellular needs. Patients who are exercising and want to optimize their cellular function level will take nutrients that support "Kreb cycle" and energy function. Finally, many patients on diets will also take a well-balanced multivitamin to ensure that they don't become nutritionally depleted.

VIII

Cognitive Techniques

W E now begin a discussion on a group of techniques that are not as tangible as those traditional patterns reviewed in the first half of this book. Yet the techniques we will now discuss are of the utmost importance in ultimately maintaining a diet for a lifetime. Permanent weight loss requires cognitive techniques—the third "R"—in which one must reorient attitudes toward a new lifestyle. To practice any of these techniques will require attitude change. This will require positively supporting a new pattern and, in a sense, making food secondary.

Rewards

As in any business, it is unwise to put all your apples in one basket. Diversification is the name of the game in big business, but it is also a critical feature in one's diet. This could best be understood by looking at the technique called "Rewards." In this technique we look to reward our daily actions. We may want to reward ourselves because the day went exceptionally well or we may want a reward because we had a really bad day.

In either scenario, the concept is to avoid using food as the reward.

Unfortunately, just as in business, when a product is a hot seller, it is hard to give it up. Food is for the most part a great reward, that is we use it to congratulate ourselves for a job well done or to comfort us after a bad day. The idea here is to diversify and find other rewards that will successfully substitute for the familiar one—food.

These substitute rewards need to be readily accessible, and they must be reasonable. Large expensive rewards like a new automobile or a vacation to Hawaii sound great but are truly only feasible once in a while. Yes, they can be planned, but there is not the same immediate gratification one gets from eating food.

For this, we try to substitute daily rewards. Some examples of more simple rewards include flowers for the table, a new book or magazine, taking in a movie or video for the VCR, buying a music CD, or merely listening to music. It may make sense also to have some rewards on a weekly basis, such as a massage at the end of the week, or a facial, etc. The major point is to diversify away from food. When one gets out from a tough day at the office, it is more adaptive to substitute one of the aforementioned rewards for food, thus enabling one to save calories in the long run. Many of these saved reward calories are wasted calories, not eaten out of hunger but more out of the feeling, "I deserve it."

Rewards also represent things that we look forward to. After a long hard day, we are tired and many times we make the error of using food as a substitute for rest. We think that by eating something we will have "more energy" and not need to sleep that much—this is obviously not the fact—indeed there is more evidence to prove the opposite situation occurs and that food makes us more drowsy. In summary then, rewards are substitutes for food that permit us to diversify our emotional response to the day into items that are enjoyably anticipated and are non-caloric. Rewards have the distinctive advantage of being able to save up their values, bank them, and eventually process them in the future.

If we look carefully, we noted that the rewards are actually substitutes for food ingestion that would ordinarily have occurred at this time of the day. This leads to another technique, which I call "Alternate Activities." Alternate activities are things that keep us busy so that we don't eat. In essence, alternate activities not only substitute cognitively, but also physically displace us from eating.

Alternate Activities

Some rewards may also be categorized under alternate activities. As an example, if I reward myself with a dance lesson, I am not eating at the time, so this fits as an alternate activity. Other rewards like the Swedish massage at the end of the week may cognitively make me give up the need for food at the moment, but since it occurs at another time, the weekend, it may not be serving as an alternative activity per se.

Alternate activities can be just about anything. If I decide to write out checks to pay my bills and not eat—then this activity is an alternate activity. It may be boring and tedious, but it still gets some of us away from food. I usually tell my patients to find both indoor and outdoor alternate activities. Doing errands, shopping, walking, and outdoor exercise all serve the purpose of alternate activities. Indoor work, such as cleaning or repairing items, serve as alternate activities. Many hobbies are both excellent alternate activities and rewards. How many of us eat while knitting or crocheting? It would be a bit messy. No one would eat while tending to their stamps or coin collections—lest they ruin the condition of the collection.

Danger in the Dark

For many of my patients, nighttime eating is a major problem. Typically these patients run themselves ragged through the day. They are workaholics fueled not by food but by high epinephrine, coffee, and anxiety. Many miss meals altogether only to get home hungry, tired, and frustrated by the laborious day. They are a set-up for abusing food.

They feel the hunger set in when their epinephrine levels start to come down. There is suddenly peace and quiet at home, and this so-called "down time" becomes dangerous, as it is a set-up for maladaptive eating. We have all experienced these kinds of down times—a quiet Saturday afternoon when there is nothing happening. It becomes an opportune time to cruise through the refrigerator or cupboard and find that leftover piece of cake or some old candy left over from Christmastime. These are the times when alternate activities become crucial. The idea is to keep busy.

Even in down time, fill the space with alternate activities. Keep busy with either a leisure activity or catch-up work. If necessary, get out of the house, go to a movie, show, or poetry reading, or be daring and exercise at home or in a gym. Exercise is a wonderful alternate activity. Indeed it kills three birds with one stone.

First, exercise replaces the time when one might eat, so it is an excellent alternate activity. Second, exercise burns calories, so it obviously helps the weight loss. Third, exercise increases epinephrine levels, and for many, this helps blunt one's appetite. Finally, exercise promotes well-being and cardiovascular fitness. It is important to plan out your activities and not go "down the garden path," resting in the lounge chair and setting yourself up for a bad food night.

Try to get right into your alternate activity. This is why those people with the gym bags at work do well. They have planned their physical activity at the gym, and they know they will be going directly there, obliterating the possibility of sabotage at home eating and not going at all.

In summary, it is alternate activities, whether they are rewards or not, that keep us busy enough to make eating food a secondary issue. The more interesting/exciting/social that alternate activity is, the better, as it is more likely to be positively supported and therefore more likely to last.

THE ASSERTIVE TECHNIQUE

There are two types of Assertive Techniques—both are very cognitive and depend on your ability to put yourself into a different paradigm. This paradigm is necessary so that you can initiate this technique. The paradigm shift is to take you, the passive patient, and put you back into the "driver's seat" as the assertive patient.

Outside sabotage is best handled by the first type of Assertive Technique. In this scenario we ask patients to make a conscious decision to be assertive. It may involve making a decision on where to go out to eat or not to eat out at all but rather to do some alternative activity. Many patients are at first embarrassed, as they feel they may be stepping on someone's toes, but upon further inspection, we see that most Assertive Techniques are either just more precise decision- making or at times merely help clarify a particular situation. That is, they are more diplomatic decisions.

One situation may involve picking out a place to dine. Suppose you are going out with two other friends. You usually keep your mouth shut and go with the flow when it comes to choosing a dining-out place. Your two friends are arguing about whether to go to a Chinese restaurant or an Italian place. Suppose now you put in your "two cents" and say, "Let's eat in a Japanese restaurant where they have that wonderful fish dish!"

Your assertiveness will now help your other two friends make a decision, and with your input, the arguing may actually stop. Even if the worst scenario occurs and all three of you argue about which restaurant is best, you are no worse off than when you didn't speak up at all, and indeed usually your opinion will, when presented diplomatically, have an impact. The key is to be heard. If not, you end up just always going with the flow.

Let's look at clarifying another position. You are at a party, and the hostess at the party is a good friend. He or she is serving everything in the world with most of the food being very caloric. You become assertive and say, "Would it be possible to have that wonderful salad on a larger plate?" Since your host is out to please, he brings forth a larger plate. The host is satisfied because he is able to please you. You are satisfied because you avoided the "greasy kid's stuff" (if you know what I mean).

Some Assertive Techniques are forceful, and though they sound abrupt, work well. Let's look first at the restaurant, you know the one where you get the basket of bread served before the meal and you know how bad a sabotage that would be. You tell the waiter, "Excuse me, sir, can you please take the bread basket away and instead bring me a tossed salad."

This sounds abrupt or even rude in certain respects, but remember a restaurant is there to *serve you* and waiters are there to please you. You are not hurting anyone's feelings by returning the bread. In the case where you are with other friends at the table, your assertive technique may involve just moving the bread to the other side of the table and then asking the waiter to bring your salad promptly so you can munch on it and not on the caloric bread and butter.

Another Assertive Technique useful at parties and social affairs is to specify a low-calorie drink and ask for it instead of getting the usual mixed drink. This again puts you in charge and avoids costly alcoholic calories. Try to be assertive at least once or twice a week. You will feel stronger about yourself and save numerous calories. Remember that assertiveness is your best method of avoiding outside sabotage.

THE DREAD OF SELF-SABOTAGE

Self-sabotage really is the most difficult cognitive technique to deal with. After all, it involves you believing you are doing the right thing. By definition, self-sabotage is a mental state that is convincing you that what you are doing is appropriate and in the end, the most useful for your well-being. In a sense, it is a break from reality, and in this sense, we can combat self-sabotage by bringing back some reality. As Mr. Spock in *Star Trek* would say, "Let's be rational."

If we look at a behavioral chain of events in which the individual has several negative behavioral links, we can demonstrate how this Mr. Spock technique works. I will call this technique the "ultimate cognitive consequence of a behavior."

We start the day off being fired from our job. This occurs after we missed the bus and arrived late at work. We feel very sorry for ourselves. To top things off, we don't get severance pay and that lousy HMO insurance is also cut. We get soaked in a rainstorm heading back home. We lose our wallet and credit card on the bus and come home with a nasty cold and a 102-degree fever. Wow, that's one hell of a day!

At 11:00 P.M. we open our refrigerator and find a beautiful cheesecake waiting there. We immediately consume one thousand calories of cheesecake and go for another slice ten minutes later. Now many of you would certainly have sympathy for this poor soul and actually say, "What the hell? Let him have it." But this is where the "ultimate cognitive consequence" is to be interceded. At the point of eating the cheesecake, this person truly believes it is the right thing to do, so he must now have himself or herself step back and become Mr. Spock.

It is best here to take a piece of paper and start jotting down the positive and negative consequences of eating that cheesecake. The positive ones may include: (1) It makes me feel better about things and it tastes wonderful. Negative consequences would include: (1) it's 2,000 calories. "Oh, my God," (2) It's full of cholesterol and bad for my health, (3) It's a weakness on my part to go down that old garden path or (4) It won't help me get my job back nor will it cure my cold.

As noted with rational input and time to look at the two different consequences, we gain rational insight and in this way take an emotional, irrational decision and turn it into a rational one. Clearly, this technique takes practice and perseverance, but it generally gives the individual a time span to think and "cool down." Even if the outcome were still to eat the cake, the increased time of thinking may have tempered the frustration and anger built up. Basically what one is doing is reassessing the situation and delaying impulsive eating.

As in any stress-induced decision, it is always best to "cool down" and introspect before acting out. Another feature of self-sabotage is that it involves negative thinking or "failure thinking." This type of self-defeating attitude basically stresses all the negative aspects of one's personality and brings out all the weaknesses. What's the use? I always fail and what does it really matter now? These are all negative set-up terms that tell the individual that he or she is unworthy of losing weight. Indeed, this becomes the dominant theme when one yo-yo diets and ultimately fails. Using the ultimate cognitive consequence rationalizes the situation and at least brings you back to a neutral zone and a less destructive one.

IX

MAINTENANCE

THE NEED FOR THE GRAY ZONE—
BATTLE 1

NOW at this point in my book, you must all be saying, "Who is this guy kidding? If I had a positive or rational attitude, I would never have gained the weight in the first place!"

In a sense, you are right. Negative thinking and persistently failing have taught you that diets don't work and that they are all doomed to fail. Naturally one is skeptical of any new technique that insists on your changing your way of thinking. But this must occur in order for you to break this long-term cycle.

Most dieters make the mistake of looking at a "diet" as all or none, black or white, win or lose. I am either on a diet or I am off the wagon. This black-or-white syndrome is further fostered by our good old friend, the scale, which tells you that you have either gained or lost weight for the week—a very black-or-white type of statement. But you, the dieter, up until this point only had the scale for proving your successes or proving your failure. To successfully keep off weight, you need to look at the subtle gray shades. As you learn those shades of gray, you will truly understand how to permanently keep weight off.

Like any battle, territory won must also be defended. In war, after each battle is won, territory captured is defended. Soldiers build perimeters, fortresses, roads, and makeshift airports to bring in needed supplies. It is only after this territory is secured that forces are able to wage the next battle and come closer to the ultimate victory of winning the war. Defending territory permanently is what wins a war and the same, as you will see, holds true for weight loss.

To understand this is to throw away the old concept of "diet" and adopt the words "change in lifestyle." The word "diet" is linked to the scale, that is "I diet, the scale goes down; I don't diet and the scale goes up" and vice versa. "Lifestyle changes" reveal all the shades of gray. If I make a subtle change in my lifestyle,I will see a subtle change in my weight. With every change there is a fine-tuning of the gray scale.

For all this to work, you need to get the words "diet" and "scale" out of your head. Think of a single subtle change in a pattern. For me, it was a change in a salad dressing from light (30 calories per tablespoon) to super light (12 calories per tablespoon). Over one year, I had a seven-pound weight loss. Now this change was extraordinarily subtle as I lost an average of 0.58 pounds per month. But the point here is that I was not dieting in the traditional sense. I had changed a pattern instead.

You, the dieter, must constantly remind yourself not to look at changes in your lifestyle as being equivalent to a traditional diet. Many patients have good intentions. They make true changes in their lifestyle and do well. Then, as time passes, they become impatient with the scale: "The weight loss is too slow;

I can't wait forever!" Generally patients who react this way are either redeveloping "scalitis" or have made lifestyle changes that are too hard to keep. I ask those patients to reevaluate what pattern changes they have made and to ask whether they feel they can commit to them for a lifetime. Many patients admit they try too quickly to make changes and in the end get frustrated and ultimately defeated by the scale. They have waged battle, taken on new territory, and are unable to defend the new boundaries, and in the end are forced to retreat.

Be very careful not to overextend yourself. Don't place time limits on how fast you must lose the weight. Don't place quantity demands on how many pounds must be lost! You need to make changes slowly, comfortably, and at your own pace.

Many of my patients have commented on how useful it is to lose minimal amounts of weight and then plateau at this early point in the weight loss period to perceive what must be done to prevent oneself from regaining weight. This ability to defend a small five-to-ten pound weight loss for some period of time, perhaps three to six months, teaches early in the game what defensive patterns one is capable of doing. "Better to test your army small scale and learn from the success or failures than to commit large forces and take the risk of total defeat."

At this point, you are probably realizing how important it is to prove to yourself that weight maintenance can occur. In my practice I have asked many of my patients to pick one or two behavioral techniques that seem reasonably easy and straightforward. I tell these patients to ignore the scale if possible and pay closer attention to their food records, telling them to lose approximately five to ten percent of their total target weight loss. Though this is a very small weight loss, it is enough to prove the defensive point of the exercise. Once the patient has achieved his or her behavioral goals and lost this minimal weight, I ask them whether they can keep off this small weight loss for the next three to six months.

Most patients ask me "am I crazy," for they want to of course lose much more weight, but those patients who take this challenge have generally been the most successful losing weight and maintaining the loss for good. This is because they have learned and accepted a subtle "gray color" in weight loss. Let's look at a scenario. Battle one. I call it "Battle of the Bulge."

The Battle Begins

My patient weighed 210 pounds and was depressed, for she had been down to 135 pounds only one year ago. She had yo-yo'd five times since age twenty-one and dieting was not getting any easier. I spoke to her at length, and she agreed to take the defensive eating challenge.

I asked her how much she would like to weigh. She said, "135 pounds or maybe 125 pounds." That was a 75-to 85-pound weight loss goal. I asked her if she was prepared to spend one and a half to two years behaviorally making changes; she thought this was a long time. I commented to her about the past *twenty-five years* of yo-yoing without success, and she agreed that one and one half years was probably reasonable. Based on my challenge, she would pick one to two techniques and achieve a weight loss of seven and a half to eight and a half pounds. At this point she was only to prove that she could successfully defend this weight loss.

The battle began. She needed first to choose the techniques that felt right for her. She chose place of eating and strict avoid-ance techniques that involved changing how she passed certain stores on her way to work. At first try she seemed to lose the weight quickly, and within only four weeks, she was down ten pounds. But then she was hit with a vacation and she was up five pounds. She was very frustrated, but I convinced her to restart. This time it seemed harder.

Week one, she was premenstrual and gained two pounds. Week two, she lost two pounds. Week three, she lost one pound. Finally, after two months she achieved a loss of 8.5 pounds. I asked her how difficult it was, and she said, "It seems doable, but I have so much more to lose."

I told her the first battle needs to be won before you go on to the next. She still had bouts of "scalitis," but over the next two months successfully stayed eight to twelve pounds below her original weight. I told her that she was quite successful with this strategy. She felt it was not enough, but this was leftover habit making her think that the more weight off, the quicker the better. I told her that the tortoise wins the race. It took some doing to get this patient off the "scalitis" kick, but with time she became desensitized to the scale and became quite successful.

THE RED ALERT OF DEFENSIVE EATING

Giving up offensive dieting takes guts! After all, the glory of dieting for many patients is that weight loss is noticed, commented on, and the "talk of the town." ("Do you know Sally? She must have lost a hundred pounds this year." "Yeah, I know, but I bet she won't keep it off." "Yeah, nobody does.") Most people who diet today are "offensive dieters." They forge ahead like tanks on a desert, watching the scale go down, conquering pound after pound only to find that just when the battle seems won, they become routed by the enemy, pull back, and regain the weight.

These patients have never set up "defensive perimeters" in their eating style. They essentially have "crash dieted."

Going into new territory requires such a different lifestyle that they could not hope to last there, even a short while. Just like in war, the farther you go into new territory, the harder it is to defend it! The enemy can cut off your supply lines, surround you, and rout you. Ultimately, you can be destroyed, captured, and imprisoned in a world of defeat, shame, hopelessness and depression. The further you go down in weight, the more vulnerable the supply lines become.

Each diet you try requires defensive patterning. Each change must be secured fully. When supply lines are formed, they must be defended and tested against the enemy. The enemy in weight loss has many "faces." Sabotage, visual cues, and lack of assertiveness can all erode your supply lines and ability to keep off weight. A defensive eating style is your only protection. Indeed, anybody who fails at a diet, fails because of a breakdown in defensive style. The good news is that with practice and a realistic battle plan, permanent weight loss is achievable.

Let's talk about defensive eating style and how to avoid being "Pearl Harbored." As in times of peace, the patient who has successfully lost weight must defend his or her weight loss. In other words, maintaining weight loss requires a continuation of basic background patterns. Just like our national defense is on guard all the time for encroaching enemies, the dieter has a series of techniques that permit him or her to keep the weight from returning.

For many, the techniques used are the same as those used

to lose the weight. Then you may ask, "What's the difference?" This could easily be understood by looking at how our nation is defended. We still have an army, a navy and an air force. They still practice all the maneuvers of warfare and battle. But in times of peace, nobody notices. In other words, just like maintaining lost weight, there is little happening on the surface. Things are peaceful and quiet, but in the background our troops are ready and alert at all times. Now on the surface there is little glory defending our nation in peacetime, yet the effort needed to keep our guards in shape and on guard is just the same. They must be ready to fight at an instant's notice. They boringly go through their maneuvers day after day with pretty much little public recognition and no glory whatsoever, yet they are always ready.

Our patients who have successfully dieted are in the same position as our troops. Whether you lose ten pounds or a hundred pounds, keeping weight off and maintaining the new weight is boring business. It is peacetime and there is no war, yet you, the patient must continue to maintain all the patterns and techniques that you used when you were in battle. It is hard to do this. It requires continually brushing up on your technique.

Though I have lost forty pounds myself, it happened twenty years ago. People who know me no longer comment on how good I look. It is "old hat" now. I am wearing the same size clothes. I look at the scale and stay within five to seven pounds of a goal weight that I defend. The glory of watching the scale go down is gone, in fact it is usually this boring pattern that sabotages so many dieters who have tried to continue to lose weight or who have lost weight and hope to maintain. Weight maintenance is a monotonous business. It is easy to just give up and "go with the flow." You, the patient, must understand that all those behavioral techniques you have learned just don't disappear with the weight loss. They become part of your everyday lifestyle and hopefully you practice them with vigor just as well as you did when initially losing the weight.

So how do I maintain the new weight without being routed? The answer again lies with our nation's defense. I set up a set of early warning signals. Some of these signals are obvious, "Gee, my pants feel tight," "My belt has to be loosened." But the most critical thing I set up is the all-important Red Alert System.

When I am in trouble, I sound this alert. My defensive perimeter is at a weight of 160 pounds. Anything below this weight creates security for me and my body. Should my weight go beyond 160 pounds, I sound the red alert. "Battle stations, battle stations!" I call on all my behavioral techniques, and I pay much closer attention to what I eat and how I behave with food. This is just like our national defense. Should an unknown aircraft fly into our territory and be captured on radar, a red alert is sounded. Our well-trained troops and air force immediately take care of the situation. Once the enemy is gone, it is peacetime again.

So we see that for weight maintenance to last, a red alert defense system must be set up. For every maintenance weight loss we are to achieve, we have a red-alert number. Even those of you who want to only lose ten pounds and keep it off will set up this red-alert number.

In a sense, every "gray shade" of weight loss that one achieves must be assigned a red-alert number. It is this number that tells you that you are in trouble and must intensify your effort with weight control. We all know that typically most patients see weight loss as black or white. They go into battle with the glory of losing lots of pounds. They think they have done well, then comes the birthday, vacation, or other celebration. They think they could just get back in control, but what happens? They develop scalitis as the numbers go up, then they feel defeated. Unfortunately, they regain all the weight, as they never set up one defensive perimeter with an early red-alert warning system.

Let's look at the patient whom we described earlier. She had lost only eight to twelve pounds in weight. She felt secure with the behavioral techniques that she had chosen to achieve this weight but had a "rocky course" even with the seemingly simple ten to twelve pound weight loss. She had to be convinced that winning even this minor battle was a major success. She hit a Red Alert two times during even this minor weight loss routine, but she still successfully defended her Red-Alert number. Remember that one year ago she had lost much more weight—seventy-five pounds! But she was immediately routed and never truly maintained her weight there. Remember that weight maintenance takes time. Before a battle is a success, you must prove you can "weather" all kinds of uncertainties. You essentially must trench in for the long haul.

Yo-yoers never do trench in; they generally regain all the weight back within two years. Remember the more the weight loss, the more vulnerable the supply lines. Keeping these behavior-modification techniques going gets rougher and requires even more practice. Many dieters in our society are unrealistic about their goal weights. They develop the "Thinderella Syndrome," thinking that if they can reach that magic number, they will do anything to keep it there. They use unsafe methods to lose unsafe quantities of weight. They set themselves up to fight a battle that can never be won. They become martyrs. "Remember so-and-so who lost a hundred pounds, wasn't that great!" "Too bad she gained it all back."

The one thing I must ask you to be is realistic—this is not a fairytale. This is your life, your health, and your well-being. Movies are about people who lose a hundred pounds in six months, keep it off, line up a modeling career, and end up on the cover of *Mademoiselle*. Real life is about successfully losing weight to a realistic number in a healthy fashion and keeping it there.

Setting up a Red-Alert number can be difficult. Should I lose ten pounds, twenty pounds or more before plateauing and defending. The answer really lies in the behavioral techniques that you choose and the intensity with which they are practiced. A better question I may ask my patients is, "How comfortable are you with the changes you have made? Can you continue these changes at this intensity indefinitely?"

If the answer is yes, I ask: "Well, what weight have you gotten down to, practicing these specific pattern changes?" The number will vary depending on initial weight starting out and whether the person is a male or female. Whatever this number is, I usually tag on five to eight pounds leeway and tell the patient this is your "Red-Alert number."

For example, John Doe weighs 220 pounds and loses 30 pounds to plateau at 190 pounds. Understanding that day-to-day weight changes vary, I ask John to give me a range of weight that he has had over the past month. He tells me he has weighed between 188 and 193 pounds. I give him my Red-Alert number of about 196 pounds. Now this 196, if hit, will tell John to sound the battle stations and get him more intense about his behavioral techniques. At a weight of 190, he has leeway to go to an event or celebrate a party and gain two to three pounds without having a major emotional breakdown. He knows he is still within a safe perimeter.

Now, after several months John came to me and said he was ready to lose another ten pounds in weight. We worked on two minor behavioral techniques. John lost ten pounds over three months and now weighed 180 pounds. We changed the Red-Alert number to 186 pounds, once again giving him some leeway to regain several pounds based on day-to-day celebrations, vacations, and lifestyle events.

This concept of leeway is critical. Imagine two nations that have warred but are now settling their differences. They set up a safety perimeter of three to four miles, a "demilitarized zone." This zone helps define a true no-war zone. If a plane or truck strays off path, they are warned but not fired upon. Our own country sets up zones, such as this, off our coast. Ten miles is the "buffer zone" before our nation would be attacked. But it is within these ten miles that the warnings are issued. These buffer zones are critical—without them skirmishes could occur continuously and constantly.

The same holds true in weight loss. Without a buffer zone of several pounds, we would never be able to eat comfortably, thinking we might be in trouble with every one or two pounds gained within the normal day. Unfortunately, people who develop scalitis while dieting are susceptible to this very problem. You see them agonizing over a one to two pound weight gain, turning their concentration away from successful techniques and toward the almighty scale. They grieve a pound gained and celebrate a pound lost. But in the end, they really go nowhere. It becomes a mental game that ultimately is destructive, sabotaging, and ends in failure.

Sounding a Red Alert requires several other important cognitive techniques. One I call avoiding failure spirals (going down the old garden path). This usually occurs when one is negative about their diet because of several failure sequences. This reminds them of past failed diets. We have all had the experience in which we catch ourselves acting a certain way due to previous experience. One gets caught up in these negative spirals and can easily break through their red-alert numbers. These negative behavioral chains are what prevents us from plateauing when we start to fail at a diet. Instead we yo-yo right back up.

You all know that feeling, "What's the use? I have gained back five of the twenty-five pounds I originally lost, this diet is impossible." Or, "Why should I be successful anyhow? I always gain it back. I am too weak to do this diet. Maybe I'll just start over again next year." It is this continuous bombardment of negative thought that drives the yo-yo'er right back up. It is called the old garden path, but for dieters it is a negative spiral cycle that leads to permanent failure and even the fear of being successful.

The Red-Alert number can help. It must be sounded, as it is the only warning signal that is concrete and real. Here is an example in which an exact number is critical. Unlike losing weight, which depends on a change in behavioral patterns, sounding a Red Alert is critically number-oriented, black and white with no gray zones. It is pretty much the opposite of what we encourage people to do when they start the diet. This is very purposeful because a Red Alert is a warning system. You can't wait for the enemy to make a major attack: Even a minor attack is an attack and must be dealt with. Appeasement does not work. It only weakens the Red-Alert number.

If I bargain with myself to move the Red-Alert number up a few pounds, I start to erode the very reason why a red alert is assigned. The Red-Alert number is a "Mr. Spock" rational number, not to be played with. If you are in a severe negative spiral and hit the Red-Alert number, you should contact your weight practitioner for immediate help. He or she will help you get back on track before you are completely defeated.

Remember if you practice behavior modification the correct way, you will only get into limited trouble because the gray zones learned are like steps that gently go up and down. If you crash-diet, it is like jumping to the top of a mountain with no steps, and when you fail, you fall all the way to the bottom. Developing a feeling of self-confidence becomes critical here.

I generally hit my Red Alert four to five times per year. When this first happened to me, it was a bit nerve-wracking. I questioned myself: "Are the techniques I practiced the correct ones; have I practiced well enough?" After I was able to conquer my Red-Alert number several times, I gained confidence in my techniques and myself. I looked at hitting the Red Alert as a test of my lifestyle and my conviction not to ever regain the weight I had lost.

TURNING THINGS AROUND

The ability to turn things around is a critical maneuver. We see it in all walks of life. In sports, the professional athlete knows how damaging negative thinking can be. The professional breaks the cycle by changing those negative feelings into a "positive rebellion." This requires a strong attitude towards one's self-confidence, but it also requires that you practice it and understand it.

It is here where the dieter must be able to turn things

around and break negative chains. "Uh oh, I am three pounds over my Red Alert. Well, I better do something." "I obviously successfully got down to this weight and I practiced my techniques successfully." "I am the one in control of my patterns." "I am the one to rebel against these negative patterns."

I call this positive rebellion. Why? Because I am basically rebelling against a negative pattern that my brain is thinking about. I am taking a leap of faith and saying "No." I will not accept the negative pattern even though this would be my natural tendency. Thus I rebel against my negative thoughts.

This is a positive rebellion because it rationally brings me back to what I really want. I see this clearly in some of my own habits. I get home late and I am tired. My body and mind say I am tired. They tell me to rest, maybe eat something. I positively rebel by going out for a jog. In the end it rationally makes sense and develops increased confidence in my ability to break a cycle. We have all done this sort of thing in our lives. It is pushing against the natural tendency toward the easy way out. It is pushing against the old garden path. Remember, travelling the old garden path just gets you back to the old garden and never lets you get to new undiscovered, fertile patterns and pathways that lead us to more fulfilling places and more fulfilling lives.

What do I do when I have broken through a Red-Alert number and find myself over a Red Alert but still in control? In other words, I have gone back on one technique. "I have lost one battle." "I have regained one shade of gray." Here it is critical that you move on and sound the Red Alert. When you lapse, don't build on it. Everybody is going to have a lapse at some point or other. The people who build on these minor failures are the ones who are more likely to have total collapse. Don't start saying, "I could have," "I should have," or "I would have." This is just ruminating old negative thoughts and enhancing them. You are lamenting about failure.

Once you identify a lapse, no matter how severe it is, the best thing to do is to move on. The less said about it, the better. Don't make mountains out of molehills. The key here is acceptance. It is human to make errors. It is more human to forgive the error. Remember, pent-up anger against yourself is the number-one sabotage to overeating and binge eating. Be kind to yourself! After all, you are the one who felt so positively about yourself. You were willing to practice and endure these new lifestyle techniques in the first place.

A positive self image is critical. People who have negative body images don't really believe they should lose—or deserve to lose—weight. Indeed, people actually start a diet because they feel positively about themselves and their ability to improve themselves. Positive body image requires that you have a realistic image of yourself—not a "Thinderella Image."

Now, we mentioned all these cognitive attributes to point out that they can either support or sabotage your ability to sound the Red Alert. People with a positive body image and self-confidence plus positive rebellious attitudes are able to handle these red-alert numbers. When these attributes are lacking, it becomes more difficult to keep to a red-alert number. Indeed, there is no guarantee that you will not get "Pearl Harbored" and caught completely off guard. The best of us can go through tough times when our priorities are simply not in weight control. It still remains critical that you are aware of the number and at least call your health practitioner so that you can be helped.

Enough said about this defensive eating mode. With

continued practice, it will become easier and easier to deal with. So what defines one's ability to successfully lose and then maintain the weight? We originally said it requires the three R's of behavior modification: Realization, Regimentation, and the all-important Reorientation. Once the patient is successful, what general patterns do we see in common with patients who are successful in keeping weight off for over two years?

One pattern in common is physical activity. When successful dieters are questioned, greater than 70 percent say they were active to a degree equal to ten miles of walking per week. Close to 50 percent did the equivalent of twenty miles of walking per week. Social support was another critical feature. If one's environment was supportive, those patients did best with weight maintenance. Support by others kept the milieu positive for these patients and made their environment favorable for weight maintenance.

Neutral partners came in second. Patients with opposing partners were the least likely to be successful in the long run and most easily sabotaged.

Low fat in the diet was a third correlation to successful long-term maintenance. Those patients who maintained a low-fat diet were again most likely to keep the weight off and maintain it.

In our practice, patients who keep daily food records and successfully sound the Red Alert have very high correlation to successfully maintaining their new weight. Indeed, keeping daily food records actually has the number-one position in potency in predicting overall success in a behavior mod weight loss program.

X

MOTIVATORS, USES, DISUSES, AND ABUSES

DO you remember when you first learned how to swim? Some of us just jumped into the water, but most of us had a "security blanket" like water wings, a tube, or a water board. By utilizing these devices, we were more confident getting into the water. We knew we would float and not sink.

Weight loss and maintenance are also learned behaviors. About 75 percent of my patients request or require a "Motivator" to get their lifestyle changes on the way. Motivators for diets achieve several positive things: (1) They give the patient a sense of security when starting a diet. Many patients lack confidence when starting a new project—just the knowledge that they will succeed at the start enhances confidence and gives the patient a positive motivator. (2) Motivators in a sense get you into the "groove" and give you positive forward momentum. Now when it comes to dieting, there are dozens of motivators—many diet books are really motivators in disguise.

Some of these motivators are unhealthy and incomplete nutritionally. They all succeed in the beginning because essentially the patient is practicing a "strict avoidance technique."

Unfortunately, what the patient doesn't know is that to be successful, other modalities must eventually be learned, otherwise the diet is doomed to fail. Water wings will get you started, but learning how to swim involves practicing a series of connecting muscular and breathing techniques.

The same is true with dieting. If you restrict yourself to just eating protein, you will have fewer eating choices and end up eating less, "Out of sight, out of mouth" theory. You will lose weight. However, if you don't learn other behavioral modes, there will come a time when you will get tired of eating protein, ultimately get bored, and of course go off the diet. Remember, "You must live a diet," not "Do a diet."

"Doing a diet" is precisely what happens to 97 percent of patients who utilize a gimmick-type diet. They all get off to a good start but have a misunderstanding of what the diet will do in the long run. Patients must remember that motivators are just that! They get you started, but the real work must still be done, and the real work involves lifestyle pattern changes via practicing patterns that last and can be supported indefinitely. Now there are many gimmick diets, all-protein diets, cabbage soup diet, macrobiotic diet, to eat carbohydrates after 7:00 P.M. and to not eat after 8:00 P.M., eat only increased fat and no carbohydrates. The list goes on and on, but unfortunately, patients don't understand that this motivator is just a gimmick and not the real diet at all.

In my practice, we initially explain these issues in detail. About 25 percent of our patients are brave enough to go right into a "behavioral mod mode" and start practicing realistic techniques right from the start. Some 75 percent of our patients ask to begin with a "motivator." About 50 percent of these patients will utilize healthy food restriction and supplements (as described below). And about 25 percent of patients will utilize medications and 25 percent will utilize healthy food and medication at the same time. We will now discuss modalities in all three groups, but it is key to remember that no matter how one starts, all our patients must engage in behavioral lifestyle changes to achieve long-term success.

Group 1 accounts for 50 percent of our patients. It is the restrictive food group with which we like to use a well-balanced diet that is easy to use and initiate. In our practice we use formulas and bars. The program consists of a protein-based beverage that is well balanced with nutrients and vitamins. This is taken two to three times a day and serves to decrease visual cues to foods. The program is presented with an outline of foods to be taken for approximately a four-week period. Meals are small and frequent, three meals/three snacks per day.

Patients are asked to fill behavioral records right from the start. Though the foods to be eaten are straightforward, we like to begin basic behavioral techniques immediately. Patients will record all basic parameters: place, time, amount, etc. Patients essentially are taken off all simple carbohydrates; white breads and potatoes are limited. The entire diet is balanced and insulin stimulation is kept to a minimum.

This helps break the increased insulin, increased hunger, binge eating cycle. Breaking the cycle is imperative, for it is the carbohydrate cycle that increases hunger and eating. We tell patients that success during this four-week period is almost guaranteed, but that long-term success is based on behavioral change and good recording of food records.

By week four of the program, most patients are comfortable enough to just continue onward with behavioral pattern changes. Some patients will extend the Motivator for a number of weeks, especially the severely overweight group. We tell patients to follow some basic rules with this diet. Patients are asked to break their eating cycle immediately on starting the motivator. If patients complain of hunger, we tell them to eat increased low-calorie vegetable products. If they are still hungry, they are allowed to increase consumption of the Motivator beverage up to five times daily.

When patients still have difficulty (this may involve those with binge behavior and compulsive eating behavior), we add an anorectic agent to the regimen. Before adding these medications, patients must have a full physical exam, lab work, and EKG. They also sign an informed consent, which outlines the potential risks of the medication.

This group essentially becomes Group 2, the restrictive food-medication group. The usual medications used are stimulant-type agents. They have the effect of increasing Epinephrine/Norepinephrine receptors. These are the same receptors that are stimulated when one is excited, the "flight or fight" system.

Patients experience a decrease in appetite and eat smaller and less frequent portions. They think less about food. The downside is some of the side effects, such as dry mouth, constipation, insomnia, and a "hyper" feeling. Most patients tolerate these agents and are able to cope with the side effects. Patients with cardiac or other significant conditions are excluded from the medication group. Patients who utilize these medications are under strict medical care. Dosages are adjusted based on lifestyle and tolerance to the drug.

For example, patients who don't get insomnia may take part of their dosage before dinner to blunt nighttime eating. When patients do complain of insomnia, the dosage is moved up earlier in the day. Patients continue to keep daily food records and practice behavioral techniques. They are told not to skip meals, even though hunger is diminished. This is because they may get used to eating with a one-meal pattern, and when the drugs are stopped, these patients classically rebound with increased daytime eating.

These drugs when used alone are not a cause for concern when it comes to pulmonary or lung dysfunction and cardiac valve dis- ease—there is no association or link. The drugs associated with these dangerous conditions have been taken off the market.

Recently several other drugs have been introduced to the market. We will discuss them briefly. These are hybrid drugs that have some features of the stimulant group discussed previously but also stimulates the Serotonin part of the brain to induce decreased craving for food. Its downside is that it can cause similar effects, as the stimulating agents including increased risk for hypertension and a rapid pulse rate. This drug may also take four to six weeks to really kick in. These drugs have not been associated with heart valve or lung disease.

A third class of agents used in practice include the Serotonin uptake inhibitor drugs. These drugs originally came out as a treatment for depression. Some of them also decrease food craving and may increase weight loss. Some have been passed by the FDA for smoking cessation to decrease the craving for cigarettes. Because of the Phen/Fen scare with cardiac valve disease, drugs have generally been less popular as a treatment for obesity at the time of this writing. Fat Blockers are completely novel drugs approved by the FDA. It causes the body to malabsorb approximately one-third of the fat eaten. It has no known internal side effects but can cause intestinal upset, including increased bowel movement, especially when the patient doesn't adhere to a low-fat diet.

Patients must also increase their intake of fat-soluble vitamins since they can be leached out by the medication. Remember that Fat Blockers do not affect the appetite at all, so patient's hunger is not changed. Some of our patients who start with a behavioral approach to weight loss may need a motivator at the start. We usually have patients try traditional pattern changes, but if they get discouraged, we may add medication to the regimen on a temporary basis to help with cravings and hunger.

This third group of patients usually understands the importance of behavioral changes but may get discouraged three to four weeks into the program, especially if weight loss is slow in coming. Medication in this group renews confidence and restimulates the patient to stay on track with behavioral techniques.

The biggest danger with all these drugs, just like with "gimmick diets," is that the patient depends more on the drug, loses weight, and never gets to lifestyle changes. These patients may develop a false sense of security and actually do well with the weight loss. They get all excited about the weight loss and forget that to continue their weight loss, long-term pattern changes must occur. Instead they veer to looking at the "almighty scale." They become intent to see the pounds shed. They continue to want the medication. They forget about food records. Ultimately this group of patients is in for a big disappointment.

Statistics tell us that most patients will gain tolerance of (get used to) the medications they are taking. This can happen as early as four to six weeks into the program. Since these patients have not practiced behavioral techniques, they become discouraged when weight loss slows. They go right down the garden path—their diagnosis is scalitis and now they are really stuck. Stopping the medications will enhance weight regain. Since they have nothing to fall back on, they are at risk of regaining all their weight.

This scenario is all too common. They have made the medication into a "magic pill" that is supposed to keep them thin forever. When this doesn't happen, frustration and depression easily can set in. These patients have misused the drugs. They fail to see the fact that the medications are only motivators, temporary boosters to get them started. It becomes imperative that any patient using a motivator has access to a strong behavioral program.

Unfortunately, many health-care providers find it easy to write prescriptions, weigh in a patient, check their blood pressure, and that's it! In this scenario, a minority of patients will succeed only to go to another program or another drug. In the worst-case scenario, patients demand to get more medication to achieve heightened weight loss. They begin increasing the dosage of medications to eke out another lost pound. Ultimately they find themselves using these drugs at higher dosages yet the weight loss is only modest. Patients may try multi-medical regimens without telling their physicians. Usually these patients develop side effects from the drug with minimal weight loss.

The ability to taper these drugs down slowly now becomes a necessity. These patients have put their health and life in danger. Many are embarrassed to tell their health-care providers that they have abused the medication. This scenario is unfortunately not uncommon. In our office we keep our eyes alert for warning signals. Patients who come in for just medication or who are asking for a brief check-up are at high risk.

When patients don't keep food records or insist on medication, it tells us that the patient's priorities may be skewed. We usually ask the patient to restate their priorities: Do you want a healthy weight loss? Is long-term weight loss important? Do you want to avoid yo-yoing? Do you really want to be on medication for long periods of time? Usually patients redevelop a sense of reality, and we can reguide them to an appropriate method of weight loss. If this chapter reminds you a bit of scalitis, it should. These very same patients who abuse medications have an extreme attraction to the scale. The all-or-none patient, the black-and-white patient is at most risk for abuse and disuse of medication.

MINI-MOTIVATORS TO GET THINGS ON THE ROAD: RECHARGING THE BATTERY

Many of our patients who have successfully practiced behavior modification can get into a slump and get close to their Red Alert numbers. Whether there has been emotional upset or perhaps just a dangerous vacation, weight gain can sneak back on. For these patients, mini-motivators can be very useful in breaking cycles. Remember defensive eating requires decisive action if a Red Alert has occurred. Cutting the cycle is imperative. For this purpose, mini-dieting with the perspective of an overall behavior mod program fits well. When a Red Alert is sounded, many of our patients will break bad habits by re-introducing the Motivator meal plan. This reorients the patient into positive thinking and breaks bad food cycles.

The secret into getting back into this plan involves two

commitments: (1) getting rid of all junk foods and simple carbo-hydrates, including refined breads and pastas (the out of sight, out of mouth theory), and (2) using the Motivator formula any time hunger becomes an issue. Some of our patients may use Motivator meal replacements four to five times daily initially to squelch hunger but after a few days, their hunger abates as insulin levels go down. Breaking a cycle thus involves getting high insulin levels down to normal or below normal. The opposite unfortunately holds true.

A diet increased in simple carbohydrates and sugars will stimulate increased insulin level and stimulate hunger, ultimately making the patient eat more and gain weight. Medication can also be intermittently used to break cycles. In this case, using the medications for a few days at a time permits the patient to break the "insulin/hunger cycle." Obviously, when cycles are broken, patients must reinforce behavioral techniques to continue to maintain weight. This becomes much easier to do since insulin and hunger are diminished.

DIETS BUILT AROUND ONE
BEHAVIORAL TECHNIQUE

Did you ever wonder how there could be so many different diets and diet books? The answer is that many, if not all, diet books are based on one or two behavioral techniques only. Many of these books concentrate on the type of foods to be eaten. Claims are made for high-carbohydrate, low-protein diet books. An example of such a book is the Dean Ornish Diet—here one eats macromolecular carbohydrates, complex in nature with a decrease in simple sugar and very low in fat. When analyzed, this diet, though healthy, is essentially restrictive. The main techniques here are: (1) strict avoidance technique, i.e., don't buy or be in front of simple sugar or high-fat foods, and (2) eat a diet high in complex carbohydrates and low in fat. These are the two techniques emphasized and employed to perform the diet.

The same exact two techniques are involved in the Dr. Atkins Diet: (1) strict avoidance—don't buy or be near carbohydrates, and (2) eat a diet high in protein and fat and low or having no carbohydrates. Note that the identical two techniques are used in both books. Essentially, this is restrictive eating with a variation on the type of food eaten.

Still other books emphasize other techniques. For example, the Rotation diet involves pre-planning and banking calories from one day to the next with food restriction. Fit for Life involves: restrictive diet, pre-planning and banking on the same diet, fruits during the day, and regular protein at night. Though patients can technically do well on any one diet, the fact that only one pattern change occurs makes it quite understandable how easy it is to fall off the diet. Just like a company that produces only one product, reliance on this product is high.

If it fails, the whole company goes out of business! Behavior mod involves some diversification of techniques. Learning to change several patterns reinforces one's ability to continue a lifestyle change. If one technique fails, there are always two or three others to back yourself up with. Companies understand the concept of diversification well. Patients who desire change must also grasp this concept.

MODULAR FOODS

Another methodology for controlling food intake and breaking a cycle is the use of modular foods. Modular foods have become quite popular recently. Considering the fast pace of work and communications, people have less time to think about and prepare foods. You essentially can do one of two things—fast food, take-out foods are one choice, but with this scenario you often end up with high fat and carbohydrate foods and poor portion control. Since you are in a rush, you tend to pay little attention to your eating style, and therefore there is an overeating of calories with weight gain.

The second and more healthy solution is to eat "modular food." Some examples include: Weight Watcher meals, Pritikin meals, and Healthy Choice dinners. These meals have several distinct advantages: (1) They are portion controlled and therefore calorie controlled. The chances are small that you would go and restart a second frozen dinner since there are time restraints and the meals are prepackaged. (2) There is a tremendous choice of foods. Healthy Choice alone has some fifty varieties. (3) There is easy storage and preparation. Just pop them into the microwave while you take a shower. (4) Many meals are actually well balanced. (5) Finally, they tend to be low in calories, some less than 300 calories per serving.

Some of my patients actually use modular foods as a motivator. If you get rid of your stored foods and junk foods and buy modular breakfast, lunch and dinner (shopping and storage technique), you will be limited to just these foods. Just get some fresh salad, eat this way for several weeks, and you will have a healthy start to your diet. You will also have an opportunity to begin behavioral techniques.

Indeed, if you do the above, you will have learned shopping and storage, strict avoidance, and portion techniques! You will also have a good start with food records, and since you are on modular foods, it would be easy to understand their caloric content and record them.

XI

THE CARDINAL RULES

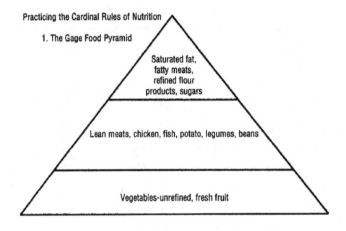

Practicing the Cardinal Rules of Nutrition

1. The Gage Food Pyramid

Saturated fat, fatty meats, refined flour products, sugars

Lean meats, chicken, fish, potato, legumes, beans

Vegetables-unrefined, fresh fruit

Follow the example and learn what to eat in three simple steps!

I was originally hesitant to include a chapter on "Food Menus and Diets." After all, the concept of my book is behavior modification, not enforced diets. However, after much thought, I decided to take my "nutritional cardinal rules" and show you how easy it is to incorporate them into your eating style.

The following is not meant to be a comprehensive compendium of diets but rather a series of examples showing you how to apply my rules. Notice I will not talk much about portion size and calorie counting, but it is obvious that portion control, especially with the high end caloric foods, is critical. So let's get started! We will do the following: a) Let's review the cardinal rules: #1. Light colored meats and animal products are better than dark colored products in the animal kingdom. #2. Refine animal prod- ucts—that is, take out the fat. Leave vegetable products untouched by human hands. #3. Vegetable products in general are better than animal products. Now let's put this to work in Diet #1 and see how the rules affect the quality of the food we are going to eat.

After this demo, I want you to notice that the intensity of the diet is actually left up to you. As you apply each rule, the diet becomes progressively healthier and less caloric in nature. You can use the rule to any extent you wish. For example, you can go to Rule #3 at breakfast, but only go to Rule #2 for lunch and perhaps only Rule #1 for dinner. This will automatically change the quality of the type of food you are eating without really thinking about how the food calorically affects your lifestyle. Realize also that there are some all-vegetable products that are quite high in calories, such as nuts and avocado. For a full description of the Cardinal Rules, see page 73 under nutritional techniques. Now let's look at other samples of diets and see how the cardinal rules again work to help you decide on the type of food that you will be eating.

Note that for each Cardinal Rule, there is a spectrum of intensity that can be "tuned" by the individual dieter.

Diet #1

Breakfast	Rule 1	Rule 2	Rule 3
Orange juice	Orange juice	Whole orange instead of juice	Orange & 1 banana
Bacon & eggs Sausage grilled with cheese	Egg white with turkey bacon, and cheese	Egg white with turkey bacon, and no fat cheese	
Black coffee	Black coffee	Black coffee	Black coffee
Lunch	Rule 1	Rule 2	Rule 3
Tuna & mayo in White pita bread with salad & fruit	White Albacore tuna &mayo in white pita bread with salad & fruit	Tuna & egg whites In natural wheat bread, salad, fruit	Salad with low cal dressing & 1 fruit, Whole wheat bread
Dinner			
Steak, mashed potato, roll broccoli, onion rings, ice cream, nuts	White chicken or turkey meat, mashed potatoes, broccoli, roll, onion rings, ice cream, nuts	White chicken or turkey meat, no skin, whole baked potato, whole wheat roll, broccoli, sliced onions, nuts, no fat ice cream	Baked potato, onion with salad, fruit or fresh nuts, whole wheat roll

Diet #2

Breakfast	Rule 1	Rule 2	Rule 3
Two eggs, bacon, ham, sausage, bagel	Egg whites with lean ham, bagel	Egg white with lean low fat ham, all natural bread 7 grain	7 grain bread, add fresh fruit
Lunch			
Fried eggplant parmigiana with French fries	Fried eggplant parmigiana with French fries	Baked eggplant made with low fat parmigiana cheese and baked potato	Eggplant ratatouille and baked potato
Dinner			
Chicken soup Deep fried shrimp, creamy cole slaw, mashed potatoes	Chicken soup, Deep fried shrimp, creamy cole slaw, mashed potatoes	Low fat chicken broth, grilled shrimp, cabbage salad, sweet potato	Vegetable soup, Tossed cabbage salad and other veggies, sweet potato grilled

Diet #3

Breakfast	Rule 1	Rule 2	Rule 3
Orange juice Ham and egg, croissant, chocolate danish, coffee	Orange juice Turkey and egg whites, croissant, chocolate danish, coffee	Whole orange Lean turkey, egg white on 7 grain bread, coffee, fruit	Whole orange, 7 grain bread, mixed fruit bowl
Lunch			
Chef's salad (roast beef, turkey, boiled egg, swiss cheese, ham on lettuce), French dressing, crackers or roll, strawberry shortcake	Chef's salad (white turkey, hard boiled egg whites, swiss cheese, lettuce) French dressing, crackers or roll, strawberry shortcake	Chef's salad (white lean turkey, egg white, no fat swiss cheese, lettuce) vinegar dressing, whole wheat cracker, strawberries	Tossed salad, vinegar dressing, whole wheat crackers, strawberries
Dinner	Rule 1	Rule 2	Rule 3
Yankee bean soup, fried crab cakes, tartar sauce, white rice, cheese cake, soda	Yankee bean soup, fried sole, tartar sauce, white rice, cheese cake, soda	Yankee bean soup (no added oils), baked sole, cucumbers, wild rice, no fat cheese cake, Perrier water or seltzer	Yankee bean soup, cucumbers, wild rice, soy cheese cake with natural bran crust, seltzer

Diet #4

Breakfast	Rule 1	Rule 2	Rule 3
Belgian waffle with butter, syrup, whipped cream, fruit on top	same	Whole wheat waffle, low fat butter buds, no fat whipped cream, fresh fruit	Whole wheat waffle with fresh fruit
Lunch			
Frankfurter on roll with sauerkraut, pickle relish, baked beans,creamy cole slaw	Turkey burger on roll with sauerkraut, pickle relish, baked beans,creamy cole slaw	Lean turkey burger on whole wheat roll, fresh beans, shredded cole slaw cucumbers	Veggie burger or tofu burger on whole wheat roll, fresh beans, shredded cole slaw, cucumbers
Dinner	Rule 1	Rule 2	Rule 3
Southern fried dark chicken pieces, tossed salad, corn muffin, blueberry pie	White fried chicken, tossed salad, corn muffin, blueberry pie	Baked white chicken, no skin, tossed salad, corn on cob, fresh blueberries	Baked sweet potato, Tossed salad, corn on cob Blueberries

Diet #5

Breakfast	Rule 1	Rule 2	Rule 3
Orange juice, French toast, powdered sugar, butter, maple syrup, sausage, chocolate donut, coffee	Orange juice, lean ham, French toast, powdered sugar, butter, maple syrup, chocolate donut, coffee	Whole orange, All natural oat bran muffin with carob covered nuts, no fat ham, coffee	Whole orange, oat bran muffin, carob covered nuts Coffee
Lunch	Rule 1	Rule 2	Rule 3
Hot Reuben's sandwich (corned beef, melted swiss cheese, sauerkraut), rye bread, apple turnover	Same except for Albacore white tuna melt	White tuna, low fat swiss cheese, lettuce, tomato, 7 grain bread, cabbage salad, baked apple	Grilled tofu, 7 grain bread, baked apple
Dinner			
Chicken and rice soup, broiled liver with onions, creamed spinach, chocolate layer cake	White chicken and rice soup, grilled veal chop, onions, creamed spinach, chocolate layer cake	White chicken with all natural rice soup, lean grilled veal chop, spinach salad, All natural muffin covered with carob	Vegetable rice soup, spinach salad, All natural muffin covered with carob

Let's look at each rule and show you an example of this. We will go from highest in calories to lowest in calories.

Rule 1: Liver is a very dark meat—Steak which is

slightly lighter—Veal, still lighter—Chicken, still lighter—Flounder, very white.

It's up to you how far to carry the change, but as you go lighter, you reduce calories. The same is true for Rule #2.

Rule 2: Refining Animal Products: Fried chicken—Broiled Chicken—Skinless Broiled Chicken—White Low Fat Chicken Slices.

Untouched Vegetables: Corn Oil—Creamed Corn—Canned Corn—Corn on the Cob.
Apple Juice—Apple Sauce—Whole Apple.

Rule 3: The highest calories in the vegetable kingdom would include: Nuts and Avocado—followed by Peas, Corn, and Squash—with the lowest being Colorful Green, Red, and Yellow Vegetables.

Though the Three Cardinal Rules are simple to under-stand, the combination of intensity and degree will help you decide how aggressively to pursue them.

XII

COMMON QUESTIONS AND ANSWERS AND MISCONCEPTIONS CONCERNING WEIGHT LOSS OR THE THINDERELLA WISH LIST

Question 1: If you eat late before sleep, you will gain more weight than eating earlier because you burn the meal off if you eat earlier. Is this correct?

Answer: Absolutely not. Calorie per calorie, time has nothing to do with how many calories are burned. What you eat is really the thing that counts. Caloric excess beyond caloric utilization will equal weight gain. The myth that eating late increases weight got started because many maladaptive eaters have high-caloric intake at night before bed. They gain weight because they overeat, and that is the whole story. One more thing, eating later is unhealthy for a different reason. You are more likely to get indigestion and heartburn when you eat late.

Question 2: If I only eat protein, I will lose weight because the bulk of calories and weight gain is caused by carbohydrates. Is this correct?

Answer: This is not correct. Generally high-protein diets also contain a fair amount of fat. Even lean protein contains four calories per gram of weight. If you eat the same number of calories of protein that you have always been eating, your weight will stay the same! If you increase your protein intake, you will gain weight. If you decrease your protein intake calorie per calorie, you will lose weight. The gimmick of high-protein diet is in part the monotony of the diet. When given only one choice of food, such as steak without the bread and potatoes, you are in part using a "strict avoidance technique" and will generally undereat quantity wise—this is one reason why people are successful with a protein diet. The problem is; can you really stay away from carbohydrates as a routine lifestyle? Most of my patients can't.

These all-or-none diets are generally too strict and many times not nutritionally sound. Different diets will contain complex carbohydrates, such as beans, vegetables and legumes, and limit the simple carbohydrates, such as bread, pasta, and dessert. Remember, it is simple carbohydrates that overstimulate insulin production and produce that vicious cycle of increased insulin, causing increased eating causing more increased secretion of insulin.

Question 3: If I eat grapefruit, citrus, and only vegetables, will I "burn the fat away?"

Answer: This is not quite correct. Eating citrus fruits and vegetables is healthy eating. The calories in whole grapefruit and oranges are relatively low, 100 to 150 kcal per fruit, pending size. Vegetables are also low in calories. However, there is no innate burning ability of these fruits. They permit your body to burn calories and since they are low in calories, you will by necessity burn fat. But a grapefruit burns no extra calories, the same being true as any other food product. There are basically low-calorie, high-fiber foods that make it easier to lose weight by nature of their ability to fill you up. There are high-density, low-fiber foods that increase calories rapidly even with only moderate capacity intake.

Question 4: After I had lost thirty pounds on a 1,200-calorie diet, I stopped losing yet I was still twenty-five pounds overweight. Is this because my metabolism shut down?

Answer: Well, yes in part. Remember, there is the "law of diminishing returns." As you lose weight, the body protects itself by decreasing its metabolic rate, thus this rate decrease can approach thirty percent decrease in basal metabolic rate. Which means, if you originally maintained your weight at 1,500-calorie intake, you would now after dieting have to eat 1,100 to 1,200 calories to maintain your weight. This is why so many dieters get sabotaged on caloric restriction diets. They lose fine, then things slow down. They develop scalitis and frustration and give up, creating the classic "yo-yo" phenomenon.

The behavior modification trainer would have initiated an exercise program that would permanently bring up the metabolic burning power. Remember, we want to keep this weight off forever. So if you are doing fine on a 1,200-calorie diet and can live with this calorie level forever, you then go to the other part of the equation and begin an increase in physical activity. Your final weight will be dictated by the level of your activity, so do what you will be capable of on a long-standing basis.

Question 5: My diet had done well, then I had gallbladder surgery and seemed to have put back on fifteen pounds. Did the surgery or operation change my metabolism?

Answer: No, but the surgery did change your lifestyle. You probably couldn't go back to your usual activities right away. You may have also increased your calories due to lifestyle change.

For example, you are home and ordering in foods. Visitors bring you food and candy as "poor you" recuperates. You don't do routine daily activities because you can't lift, etc. Even a lifestyle change of several months can severely disrupt the diet. Preplanning techniques are critical here. Many patients play the "sick role," which they think entitles them to food ad lib. Beware of internal and outside sabotage here.

Question 6: I have "yo-yo'd" many times, losing and
    regaining weight. Didn't this ruin my metabolism so
    that I will have a much harder time losing again?

Answer: Theoretically when you lose weight, you lose
    both fat and protein. When one follows a sound
    diet, three-quarters of the weight loss is fat; twenty-
    five percent or so is protein. But rapid loss "crash
    diets" cause the body to lose more protein. When
    this occurs over and over again, your body compo-
    sition will have less protein (muscle) and more fat.
    Remember, it is the "muscle-protein" that burns fat.
    Fat cells just store fat and burn little energy. Thus the
    "yo-yoer" is somewhat less efficient at burning calo-
    ries. The answer here is to never "crash diet" and to
    build up protein (muscle). This is done by exercising
    and physically putting your body into better shape.
    Exercise works the muscle and the muscle essentially
    burns fat as fuel.

Question 7: It seems as if the minute I stop dieting, I
    begin to regain the weight. Do I have to diet the rest
    of my life?

Answer: This is a matter of definition. The average
    American looks at a diet as a temporary, sometimes
    torturing adventure. After "doing the diet," he or she
    then looks forward to getting back to his or her usual
    lifestyle, which has not changed and leads to regain
    of weight, usually to the original baseline weight.
    The behavior mod person changes patterns—hope-
    fully permanently and therefore "lives the diet." The
    bottom-line answer is yes—our definition of diet

is hopefully for good. That is why the concept of reorientation is so critical here. It is the essence of behavior mod and defensive eating style. It is the opposite of the Thinderella Syndrome. Right now, 97 percent plus dieters are Thinderellas. Hopefully, the techniques in this book will change that figure substantially.

Question 8: Do over-the-counter diet pills work?

Answer: Most of these pills are weak sympathomenes with other additives such as caffeine or Ephedra and herbal sympathometic added in. People take these pills in an uncontrolled manner and are not medically monitored; thus the danger of stroke and hypertension are very real. Even when taken correctly, they may only temporarily inhibit appetite. Most patients don't practice the behavioral techniques needed, and over time the pills stop working. Thus, the average patient is not successful with over-the-counter medicines.

Question 9: Many times when I am dieting, several weeks can go by when I see little or no weight loss or even put on a pound. I am exact with my diet and style of eating and exercise. What happened?

Answer: Several things may be going on. First, remember that your body is 60 percent water, which means that a small shift of water, either excess or depletion, can shift your weight several pounds in either direction. Especially in women, pre-and post-menstruation, weight can vary four or more pounds.

This premenstrual weight can be very sabotaging to women. I have had several patients on all-formula diets actually gain a few pounds when they were premenstrual. They clearly were upset and really needed to understand this water concept. Usually the week after menstruation, there is a loss of water and the weight goes down more than expected. Because of the sabotage effect of water weight, I encourage all patients, even those on pure formula diets, to do accurate daily food records. This clearly helps lessen the sabotaging effect of water shifts. At times water retention may decrease weight loss for several weeks at a time. This can be frustrating but the "real weight will come off in time." These bouts of water retention can occur secondary to increased sodium intake. Remember sauerkraut and sour cucumbers are low in calories but high in salt. These foods clearly demonstrate that a low-calorie food can cause water weight gain. Patients who record food records know that the caloric content of sour pickles and sauerkraut are low so they know the weight gain is water weight not "real weight." Remember the whole danger here is that patients who don't trust their food records or don't do them could develop "scalitis" and sabotage the whole effort.

Finally there are patients who have lost a lot of weight and then "plateau" in their weight loss. In part this is a fluid shift situation as above. It may also be caused by the decrease in metabolic rate that kicks in after one has dieted for a while. It is at this time when exercise becomes much more important.

Remember that there are two ways to lose weight: one is restricting calories, the other is increasing activity. Also remember that at the beginning of a diet, caloric restriction has its biggest punch. With the "law of diminishing returns" occurring as one continues to diet, the effect of caloric restriction diminishes. Exercise, on the other hand, becomes more important with time for two reasons: 1. It becomes easier to exercise as your body weight goes down, your activity levels get better, and you are gradually increasing the level. 2. Exercise is the only healthy way to combat the body's decrease in metabolic rate that occurs when dieting. Exercise speeds up the metabolism.

Question 10: Is it true that eating six meals a day will help me burn fat?

Answer: Eating small frequent balanced meals is a healthy thing to do. In fact most very obese individuals eat large meals, usually at night and they typically skip breakfast! In any event "burning fat" occurs because of a negative calorie balance. That is obtained in only two ways: 1. Eat less than you burn per day, or 2. Increase your activity to burn more calories than you eat.

Question 11: What is the optimal percentage of protein, carbohydrates, and fats to lose weight the quickest way?

Answer: Though the exact numbers here seem to always change, general principles can be followed. Twenty-six percent of fat or less, with most fat being unsaturated, is ideal. The fewer simple carbohydrates, the better, but complex carbs: vegetables, legumes, beans, fruit, etc., are good for you. The average adult only needs 40 grams of protein to survive, but 60 to 75 grams seem optimal.

Barry Sears described the "Zone Diet" of 40 percent carbohydrate, 30 percent fat, 30 percent protein and this seems fairly close to being just about right, but remember, too much food, even all protein, will still put on weight! Also remember that each person's diet needs some individualization. For example, the forty-mile-per-week jogger will need some increase in the carbohydrate percentile. The obese pre-diabetic patient will need fewer carbohydrates and fewer simple carbohydrates. Your health professional can guide you in general. Remember to follow the three Cardinal Rules of Nutrition!

Question 12: Does your ability to process sugar directly affect the balance of protein, fats, and carbohydrates that you eat when you are trying to lose weight?

Answer: Sugars are generally similar to simple carbohydrates in terms of metabolism. That is, a piece of candy and a purified piece of white bread are treated in a similar fashion. If you eat a piece of candy, then calorie for calorie, leave out a piece of white bread or a pasta dish. To create balance in your diet, always make this kind of trade-off. Remember, the fewer simple carbohydrates, the better off you are with your diet.

Question 13: Since everyone is all hung up about no carbohydrate diets, why should people eat carbs at all?

Answer: There are several reasons to eat healthy carbohydrates (complex carbohydrates) in your diet. First, the carbohydrates provide us with an energy source. They are still less caloric gram for gram compared to other energy sources such as fat.

Secondly, complex carbohydrates are our main source of fiber. This is critical for correct digestive function and correct bowel habits. A lack of fiber is considered to be a major cause for digestive ailments in Western civilization. Colon diverticulosis (pockets), colon cancer, and hemorrhoids are all thought to be in part caused by lack of fiber.

Third, complex carbohydrates found in fibered foods, such as beans and vegetables, help fill us up. Complex carbohydrate foods are generally bulky and relatively low in calories. Celery, salad, and legumes all contain small to modest amounts of complex carbs in their cell walls. These foods are also generally rich in antioxidants, vitamins, and minerals; all good for you!

Question 14: What is the cause of cellulite? Can it be cured?

Answer: In general, cellulite is the lumpy, bumpy fat and collagen tissue under the skin. It occurs with increasing weight gain and may also be partially hormonally induced by changes in insulin level and female hormone changes. Lipodystrophy (reabsorption of fat and fat deposition in an uncoordinated fashion) will produce the cosmetic outcome of

cellulite. The best cure is not to ever develop it.
An ounce of prevention is worth a pound of cure
(pardon the pun).

The reality is that once the fat deposits occur, only
plastic surgery and liposuction are the answer. Weight
loss may help the condition by reducing the size of
the fat deposit. Certainly the magical gimmicks out
there are not the answer. Pounding on cellulite with
a large paddle only creates edema and tissue damage,
which temporarily covers up the lumpy, bumpy look.
Medication and fat burners have never been successfully proven to get rid of cellulite.

Question 15: When one gets older, does the metabolism
slow down? Should I weigh more at age fifty than I
weighed at age thirty?

Answer: Interestingly, one's metabolic rate stays pretty
much constant throughout adult life. Not until the
age of seventy or higher does it seem to decrease, and
this may be in part due to a decrease in muscle mass
that occurs at this age. The reality is that as people get
older, they become more sedentary. The proverbial
"beer belly" develops due to the lack of activity and
the continuous eating of similar amounts of calories.
People become busy with their careers and families.
They change their lifestyle and thus the midlife mid-
drift occurs. The answer is to stay active and continue
to eat healthy simultaneously.

Question 16: What is an ideal amount of weight to lose
per month?

Answer: Generally one percent of body weight loss per week is a safe amount. However, remember not to set goals based on specific weights. Based on two hundred pounds, a patient can safely lose up to eight pounds per month. However, we advise only using the number to avoid losing faster than this rate. When a patient loses weight too fast, it is an indication that protein loss will exceed the twenty-five percent ideal amount of weight loss. This is dangerous on several accounts: first, you will lose too much protein. This represents your body's healthy weight, muscle and organs. It is the muscle and organs that burn calories, so you will reduce your ability to lose weight over time because you will burn fewer calories. Second, rapid weight loss over time has been associated with dangerous health consequences; sudden death and cardiac arrhythmia (irregularities) were well known to plague those individuals who were on 500 calories and water fast-type diets in the 1960s. Protein malnutrition is therefore a very dangerous thing.

Question 17: I have been told that drinking eight glasses of water will speed up my weight loss. Is this true?

Answer: This is partially true in an indirect way. Water itself has no calories, but it does take up space! This means that if water is in your stomach, there is less room for caloric food and you will eat less. Drinking water itself is healthy. Besides maintaining fluid balance, it improves intestinal function and permits the body to clear toxic wastes through the kidney.

Question 18: I have been told that exercising before or
    after a meal will burn off the meal. Is this true?

Answer: That all depends how many calories you are
    eating. A 300-calorie meal can be burned off by
    exercising the equivalent of 300 calories, for example
    three miles of walking. Timing of the exercise right
    before or right after a meal may have some subtle
    added advantages. For example, some people who
    intensely exercise may actually blunt their appetites
    for a while and therefore decrease hunger and eat
    less during the mealtime. There are some studies that
    suggest that you will burn some extra calories by exer-
    cising close to mealtime. However, most experts agree
    this added burning is minimal and amounts to less
    than ten calories per day. Remember that you should
    exercise when it is comfortable for you to do so.
    Some people get symptoms of stomach upset when
    they exercise too soon after eating. Try to use your
    exercise as an alternate activity and calorie burner.
    Don't worry about the timing.

AFTERWORD

THE THINDERELLA REALITY TEST

SO, let's now look at the new Thinderella. She or He is a person with confidence and self-esteem. Having practiced lifestyle pattern changes, Thinderella has successfully achieved a healthy, realistic body weight. Thinderella does a daily food record and pre-plans all meals. Thinderella eats slowly and at the table. Thinderella knows how to "bank calories" for those big palace balls that are thrown with frequency. Thinderella knows how to exercise realistically and frequently. Thinderella doesn't overdo it at the ball, rather he or she eats with moderation on small plates that are served in the classic European fashion.

Thinderella is assertive and tells her two step-sisters to "bug off" and therefore goes to all the palace balls without magical pumpkin carriages. Thinderella does not expect magic things like a perfect prince or princess. Instead, Thinderella knows that all good things are worked for and earned. Thinderella has perseverance and patience. Thinderella is not sabotaged easily. It takes a lot to interfere with his or her habits. By using the well practiced habits of behavior modification, Thinderella knows that even if there is a slight "fall back" in patterns, there is nothing to be flustered about. Rather it is looked at as an expected human error—after all we are not white-and-black or all-or-none type perfectionists. Thinderella rolls with the punches and knows boundaries well. Thinderella can defend himself/ herself because Thinderella has truly re-oriented his or her lifestyle for good. We have a lot more faith in the new Thinderella who will look at the world realistically and maintain a weight because this is the lifestyle practiced.

We congratulate the new Thinderella because he or she will earn the crown of a healthy lifestyle.